I NEVER RANG THE BELL

I never rang the bell

A MEMOIR

Andrea Leigh Ritcey

Life isn't about waiting
for the storm to pass;
It's about learning
to dance in the rain.

— Vivian Greene

CONTENTS

PART TWO

PART THREE

Message from the Author

For years, I was afraid. Afraid to speak up, afraid to question, and certainly afraid to contradict anyone. I managed like this well into adulthood. Slowly I evolved, and, just when I thought life was as good as it possibly could be, unthinkably, I was diagnosed with cancer. Forced to find my voice, to advocate for myself and to meet conflicts and challenges head on, *I Never Rang the Bell* is a memoir that uniquely shares my shocking experience and the enormous personal growth I gained during this highly pivotal year.

My hope is that my journey will inspire you; to demonstrate how the power of optimism can get you through some of the worst of times. If life has not already knocked you to the ground, at some point, it may still. These moments are part of being human. How do we cope in those very trying times? How do we feel joy when life unfolds in such catastrophic ways and more importantly, how do we recover? The answer lies within and this is where the true work begins. I encourage you to consider that life isn't about the final destination; the joy very much needs to be in the ride.

In full "survival mode," I found myself desperately searching for answers to all things cancer. Utterly blind-sided by how it completely took over my life, *I Never Rang the Bell* is my journey from beginning to end; the day I received my diagnosis, the surgery and staging, the various treatments and the inevitable PTSD. Along with that, a complete rollercoaster of "feels" with hilarious moments, entertaining childhood memories, a love story between husband and wife, dark moments of despair, contrasting moments of joy, some nods (of course) to my 200-pound English Mastiff, and, most importantly, it's about finding my inner strength. My story is compelling and, at the risk of sounding cliché, you will laugh and likely cry but I promise I've kept the worst of the gloom and doom to a minimum.

Admittedly, some of the chapters were very uncomfortable and quite personal to discuss and I found myself questioning, *do I really want readers to know I experienced this?* Upon reflection, I felt the knowledge one gains through my words overpowers the humiliation of my tell-all. And so I prevailed; subsequently throwing all privacy out the window with total, reckless abandon.

We know that cancer can be intensely scary, utterly devastating and all encompassing. Surprisingly though, I learned it can also be strengthening, empowering, uplifting and can guide one to new heights both in self discovery and in more meaningful relationships. While at my lowest, I realized that determination, tenacity, grit, humour and a positive outlook are some of the most prominent qualities needed to manage cancer and more generally, to survive life. I am living proof that the power of the mind matters when it comes to dealing with a major diagnosis or crises, severe trauma or an intense, debilitating disease. It is my intention through my story that you will be inspired to grow in strength in order to manage your own situation when you find life so very tough to manage; be it an illness, or another aspect in your life.

If my memoir has found you with no cancer connection, may you see this book for all that it offers on a different level; the take away being that you learn to meet challenges head on with bravery, inner strength and with as much grace as you can find. Seeing things optimistically (even in the worst of life's moments) can greatly influence how you feel and how you manage throughout your life. If practiced, you can find humour in even the most trying of times.

In addition, my story is also intended for partners and care givers, relatives and friends to know first hand what their loved one is experiencing and feeling and how best to support them. This book demonstrates what a healthy partnership can look like.

No matter where you are in your life's journey, it is my sincerest hope that you come away feeling new found strength; that you can allow yourself some growth, that it's ok to "clean house" in interpersonal relationships and that quite frankly, to manage an ongoing debilitating disease or any other intense disaster, takes a village and it's okay to lean on people for that support.

Our vast, mystical universe is ours to learn from. It speaks to us if we gently ask and quietly listen. Lastly, *I Never Rang the Bell* is about learning to connect to your inner voice. The universe does and will speak to you and can guide you to your highest good. You just have to be open, be ready and to allow it.

And this is where I leave you. To ponder, to hope and to believe.

Love,
Andrea Leigh Ritcey

PROLOGUE

I n the end, I never *did* ring the bell. Oh now don't get me wrong . . . I'd planned on ringing the absolute shit out of it. I'd invite my family and friends; we'd eat cake and take pictures and pay a tribute to the nurses and . . . you know . . . the whole nine yards. I'd wear my soft pink cashmere poncho, my camouflage leggings and my bright, bubble gum boxing gloves. I'd do it all up "fancy-like;" more extravagant than a designer float in a Macy's Day Parade. I'd go *completely* all out; and maybe at the end of the party I'd shoot off fireworks bigger than the Fourth of July.

I absolutely couldn't wait for that day; for months it was really my only focus. But in the end, none of that hoopla mattered anymore. I just wanted to have . . . silence.

PART ONE

1
DAY ZERO

"It's cancer, isn't it."

It wasn't really a question, rather a flat-out assertion; a bold, in-your-face challenge. I sat bravely staring at this virtual stranger three feet away from me, who was about to tell me some life-altering news. It didn't matter that she hadn't yet spoken; her face said it all. What seemed like more than a billion painful seconds passed by, and yet I waited. I waited and waited, and I waited some more.

The walls around me slowly started to close in. The air became stale. I became fidgety and yet at the same time, strangely calm. The fact that she hadn't yet met my eyes with denial allowed me on some miniscule, cellular level to slowly allow the potential to sink in.

The stranger looked back at me, this specialist. This . . . gynecological-*oncologist* specialist. She scratched her head and then double-checked her file. I watched her take in a slow, deep breath, perhaps preparing herself to deliver the devastating news, or perhaps, assessing me, my mental strength. Finally, she replied.

"Yes. Yes. It is cancer."

The words hung in the air briefly and then reached my brain with electrifying speed. BOOM! Just like that. A smack in the face with a giant Bugs Bunny anvil: "DING!" The force of it hit my head just like in the cartoon, an instant concussive egg rising up three inches like a stalagmite, birds chirping and flying around. Somewhere deep within my body, I felt myself start to go numb. Stunned, I looked back at this woman and just . . . accepted the news. I didn't cry. I didn't gasp. I just sat there with my COVID mask and blank eyes, processing this new information.

I had told my husband to wait in the car. I do confess, I *was* expecting to hear the most awful news, and I didn't really know how I would take it. I didn't want him to see my reaction in case I totally lost it. (How can one anticipate how they will react to such news?) Even though hearing the diagnosis out loud came as a shock, deep down, I knew I had cancer. I had had this nagging inner voice in my head for months. I couldn't shake it. Each time I had a quiet moment to myself, this voice would speak to me: *You have cancer, go get checked.* I questioned that voice; cancer didn't run in my family. Nevertheless, my inner voice persisted, and I made sure to pay attention. I had learned a very long time ago that when your inner voice whispers, then talks, and then starts yelling, you *need* to listen—it's your intuition forcing you to act. Mine kept me up at night.

And so, as odd as it seemed, this appointment for me, this "meeting," was simply an outward confirmation from a medical professional. I suspect that's why I didn't pass out, or scream, or start hysterically crying.

"Look," she said, "I'm as shocked as you are. You are a young, vibrant, healthy-looking woman. This type of cancer is highly unusual for a person of your age. But the good news is, under the microscope, these cancer cells look pretty decent. They are not all misshapen and ugly." I stared at her as she continued. "So, it's likely just a quick hysterectomy, and then you're good to go. Okay?"

Eyebrows raised and pen tapping, she said it like it was a cake order for a wedding. I felt my ears start to ring as she handed me all sorts of papers: the yellow one was for the Nova Scotia Cancer Centre, the pink one was for blood work, a white one was for the family doctor. "Okay?" she said again, sort of loudly. I realized I had heard her saying okay several times before I clued in that she was still talking to me.

"Okay what?" I asked. My brain simply wasn't computing.

She looked at me quizzically. "Have you heard anything I've said for the past five minutes?"

"Yes. Yes, I'm good. Thank you," I lied. In fact, I had missed *everything* she'd said. But what did it matter? I was sure I'd receive numerous papers and phone calls in the next several days, and I figured I could take in then what I needed *when* I needed.

The doctor left. I got up. I have to say, even though I was both shocked and stunned at the confirmation of my own prediction, I handled the news rather well. That life-changing moment was comparable to one of those times when one asks, "Where were you when you learned the news that so-and-so died?" or "Where were you when 9-11 happened?" The mind-blowing, shocking, brain-numbing type of news that literally stops you in your tracks and makes your blood run cold. The sort of news that, at best, you can turn to someone you know and hug them instantly and cry, if need be. The sort of news that stays with you for *the rest of your life*. But there I was, by myself, taking it all in, like a champ. Oddly, it was as if I was having an out of body experience; I was standing there, looking at this red-haired woman, thinking, *Damn . . . she's strong. So calm. She's . . . amazing.*

Then my perspective changed, and I was back inside myself, thinking, *Holy, girlfriend, you just received horrible news and you just learned something—you can handle this. You can do this. You don't need to fall on the floor in hysterics, terrified. You are contained. You are in control. You are . . . powerful.* And in that moment, the security I felt in knowing that I was going to look after myself almost felt like I had two personalities, two perspectives. I was the fighter, the caregiver, the warrior, but I was also the one who had fallen prey to this horrible disease.

In the midst of all this self-realization, which took mere moments, was a life-altering awareness—I can cope. I will get through this; I will survive and I don't need anyone to pull on my arm to keep me from jumping off the bridge. I didn't know that I possessed this kind of resolve, this determination. Oddly, amongst the strong emotions surfacing that day, I felt . . . proud.

I texted my husband that I was finished the appointment and for him to pick me up. He called me as I was leaving the examining room.

"Well?" he inquired. "How did everything go?" There was an urgency to his voice. He sounded odd.

"Not good," I replied, in a voice I had never heard before that moment. I didn't even recognize it. It sounded so completely defeated, scared; like a person in shock.

"Okay," he said, "I'll be out front in two minutes."

As I dazedly walked down the long hospital corridor, I noticed that the demeanour of the nurses at the station had changed. I suspect the doctor, moments before, had told them the news, that she'd dropped the hammer and delivered the blow.

"See ya," I said. Their faces, full of empathy, sadness, and awkwardness, left me feeling uneasy. Clearly they knew much more than me about the hell I was about to go through—much, *much* more.

2

A ZOMBIE ON GRAVOL

I got in the car and my husband looked at me. "What's happening?" he asked, trying to maintain his self-control.

In a pinched, slightly angry sounding voice, I replied, "Drive. Just . . . drive."

We had to get out of the busy hospital parking lot, and there were way too many pedestrians, bikes, taxis, buses, and ambulances crowding us in. We dodged several people and several obstacles, drove into a neighbouring street, and Mike pulled over. I sat in silence as he stared at me. I took a deep breath, turned, and looked straight at him. As he looked back at me, I could tell he had figured out that the news we both had truly feared was now confirmed. I said it out loud for the first time. "I have cancer."

The words just sat there. It was such an abnormal thing to say. I had to actually say it three more times before I could understand the statement to be true. Mike looked at me like I had just spoken a foreign language; he was equally shocked. If you were to add a shot of scared and a cup of angry to a bowl full of confusion, you might start to understand what we were feeling. To put it simply, we had no words. Too shocked to cry and too scared to speak, we just sat there. And so, in silence, we began our drive home.

As we made our way, the hospital called and wanted to book blood tests. Given that we lived in a little coastal village forty-five minutes away, I politely explained, "It's an hour and a half drive for us round trip. How soon can we do this?"

They quickly replied, "Can you come right now?" So, with no discussion whatsoever, Mike whirled the car around and drove us right back to the hospital.

This time, as I walked through those doors, I held the knowledge that I was a person living with cancer. I immediately had a different perspective. How many other normal, healthy-looking people were walking around in front of me with a cancer diagnosis? I had assumed all able-bodied, healthy-looking people were just that; healthy. I was in such a complete daze, I walked into a concrete post. "Watch it!" a man said, chuckling. He then looked quite shocked when he saw my face—empty, blank, stunned.

My mind was racing. How could I *possibly* have cancer? I looked healthy, with auburn hair halfway down my back, youthful skin and a sparkle in my eyes. I was a plump fifty-one, the typical perimenopausal body (well, maybe I was a little chubbier than plump), but I walked with confidence, strength, and good posture. In my mind, I couldn't have cancer—I didn't look the part. I was not gaunt, thin, sickly. I thought people living with cancer were pale, skinny, ill-looking. I was robust. Big bosomed. I golfed. I sailed. I walked our two-hundred-pound mastiff roughly fifty kilometres a week. Getting a cancer diagnosis (even though a voice in my head had me worried for months) was, nevertheless, still completely surreal.

I located the lab for blood work. A friendly lady at the desk smiled at me and softly explained, "We are a little behind, but we will get to you soon." I sat there in silence taking things in, and then out of nowhere, with no warning at all, massive, uncontrollable, shaking sobs burst from my body. I was again all by myself, as parking was problematic and I had told my husband that I'd only be a few minutes.

I kept having to rein in my sobs as people passed through the waiting area. Finally, after about forty minutes, I flagged down a nurse and in between my quiet outbursts I asked, "Do you know how much longer this will be? I just learned I have cancer. I'm trying my hardest to keep myself together but I need to get out of here. I want to go home and hug my dog."

Her face immediately turned sad. "Oh my gosh," she said quietly, "I am so, so, so sorry." She gave me a solid hug. A stranger, hugging me. Other than Mike, the first with whom I shared my news was a stranger.

Not two minutes later I was sitting in the blood collection La-Z-Boy and the technicians were working hard at getting some blood out of my very small veins. I was still in shock, snivelling and staring into space like a zombie on Gravol, trying to process what this news meant for me, my family, and what kind of journey lay ahead.

"Okay, all done!" The blood collection nurse smiled at me as she placed my hand firmly over the cotton ball covering up the point of entry. "Good luck with everything," she sang. She seemed so chipper and happy, carefree and oblivious to my zombie-like state. The contrast in our demeanours and my silence, my inability to even respond, was pretty stark.

I numbly got up, walked again down the long hospital corridors, through the lobby, and out into the blinding sunlight.

Endometrial adenocarcinoma. That's the type of cancer I'd been told I had. A mouthful to say of course, being a whole twelve syllables long, but I eventually learned it and committed it to memory. Waiting in the car, Mike had read the papers from the specialist and had done some research while I was getting the blood work. As I got into the car, he started pumping out stats. "Okay. Seventy percent of people at this age have this percent likelihood of survival," blah, blah, blah. I was so completely dazed; I couldn't understand how he knew all of this. I barely recall the drive home. We could've flown in a spaceship for all I knew.

As we pulled into our driveway, I tried to process the events of the morning. This was an enormous, staggering diagnosis. It had already been a crazy week for us as we had just moved into a beautiful new home only four days earlier and were completely knackered from unpacking a gazillion boxes, still with a gazillion more to go. My mind spinning, it quickly flashed back to our night before; Mike and I had been sipping wine and relaxing on the couch. Looking around at how much we'd unpacked and organized, I felt deeply satisfied and full of joy. "I feel like we are living in a dream! I can't believe we actually live on the ocean in this beautiful log home! I can't believe how happy I am. I am the happiest I've been in a very long time." I'd kissed his cheek and smiled. "Life is finally coming together for us." Well. That didn't last long. We had had only three days of bliss.

Even just this morning, I had woken up still feeling immensely joyful. I had decided to take a break from the brutal schedule we had set, to venture out on the property. We were trying to get the house ready for a house-warming and brunch for our family two days from now. I had needed fresh air and some new motivation, as I was a bit overwhelmed with our ambitious undertaking.

I put on my sweater and boots and walked outside to the glorious fresh ocean air. At the front of the house, large wooden stairs made from railroad ties led to an upper field that I had yet to even explore. I decided to venture up to see what was what. I was impressed and excited as I climbed each step, and I noticed more and more shrubs and unique rocks on the property. When I finally reached the top, I turned to look at the view below, and I gasped as I took in the ocean scene in all its glory. It truly looked like something out of a movie. I stood atop the long, grassy slope of our hill and looked down below at our sturdy, secluded, safe haven. Taking a photograph in my mind, I freeze-framed the log home, the ocean with its crashing surf, the sandy cove, and the towering, seventy-five-foot rock wall on the right. There was an island far off in the distance. The view was simply mesmerizing.

I stood there, smiling. *Wow!* I thought. *This is surreal.* I had actually found my Utopia. I stayed on top of that hill for several more minutes, watching the waves crash, the trees gently sway in the wind, and the occasional seagull rush by.

I still had much to unpack, so I eventually continued on my brief but happy exploration. I walked a little farther and came across the beginning of a path. Curiously I followed it and, to my delight, discovered a gold-coloured Buddha with a giant belly and a jovial, dimpled face, sitting on a little hill. The sun was shining down on this simple statue, and I laughed out loud and said, "Well hello, Buddha! Nice to see you!" I waited to see if he would reply, but he didn't. I continued on the path and came across two gigantic stones, each about four feet high. My body suddenly felt tingly with excitement and energy. I stood there, intrigued, and gently placed my hands on top of their cold, smooth surface. I closed my eyes and tried to feel their strength. I tried to imagine the storms they had weathered and wondered about the years they had existed.

I stayed in that position for several minutes, standing in between the stones, one hand placed on each, in my silent world of intrigue and joy. Eyes still closed, I breathed slowly, deeply, in and out. Oddly enough, I felt rejuvenated. It was as if the stones had given me new-found energy. Amazed, I realized they'd also given me the grounding I hadn't known I needed; I gently gave them a parting pat. "Thank you," I said to the stones, and I continued on the path. As I walked, my eyes caught yet another intriguing figure in the woods. I approached it, thinking, *What am I seeing? A baby?* My steps quickened as I discovered a small, bald figure. It was holding a book, kneeling on another mossy hill. As I arrived, I realized what I was looking at. "Oh!" I exclaimed out loud. "It's a monk! How perfect!" The fat, jovial Buddha I had met moments before was perfectly balanced by the skinny, wise-looking monk holding a book and meditating. "Hello there, sir," I said to the monk, instantly loving it. It was a unique statue and reminded me of the importance to take time to reflect and to sit quietly; to focus.

Finally, the path came to an end. I could walk to the left to connect back to our driveway, or to the right to go a little farther off property. For some reason, I felt compelled to go to the right. As I slowly walked along, I felt an odd sensation; it was as if electricity was in the air. Again I felt tingly, zingy. I came to an open field and walked a few more steps and then abruptly, I stopped. I stood very still and had the urge to close my eyes again; it was odd for me to feel this way. *Why am I standing here in a field with my eyes closed? What am I feeling?* Moments later, I felt my arms slowly rise up in front of me and then my hands turned over, allowing my palms to sit open, chest level, parallel to the sky. *What is happening right now?* I hadn't ever really stood like this before, but my body had led me to this space, and unconsciously I came to this position. I stayed like that for several minutes, meditative, breathing deeply, palms up and eyes closed. I felt stuck to the ground; my feet didn't want to move. My body was arched over a bit, not completely upright and it very gently swayed. *Was it the wind? Or was it because my feet had positioned themselves in a way to receive energy from deep below the earth's surface?* To this day I will never know or understand the why's of that fascinating moment, but I came away feeling incredibly energized and joyful, as if all things were right in the world. I'd stayed there for a good five minutes, almost trance-like and again, like my experience with the stones, I felt rejuvenated. And just as it had inexplicably happened, it also was inexplicably over. Feeling satisfied and ready to continue on with our move, I returned to the house, slightly perturbed but mostly excited to get to know this magical, fascinating space.

My phone rang as I walked inside. It was the hospital calling to say the results were in from my biopsy a few weeks before and that I needed to come in to discuss.

"Can't you just tell me the results over the phone?" I pleaded. "We live all the way out in Peggy's Cove, and we are in the middle of unpacking."

"No," the voice paused, "we don't give results like this over the phone."

And so, with a sick, awful, spiralling feeling, I hung up the phone and nervously turned to Mike, "We need to go."

3

DOG TEARS

The drive in, the appointment, the news, the blood work, and the drive back out had all taken just under three hours. It's incredible to think how in the space of that very short time, our lives were forever changed. We went from feeling glorious and peaceful, excited and full of hope, to completely gutted, devastated, numb, scared, and in shock. As we walked through the front door of our new home, surrounded by cardboard boxes and random items, we simply stumbled to the couch and sat down hard. We sat in silence for quite a while and just stared at the floor. Large plastic totes were piled ten feet high and a planned brunch for eleven people, less than forty-eight hours away, was looming.

"I think I need to cancel the brunch," I said. I was back to unpacking again.

Mike came over and wrapped his arms around me. "Let's talk about this. If we cancel, people are going to wonder what's up."

"Tell them we have COVID," I pleaded. *How on earth would I keep myself together?*

"No. If we do that then no one can visit us for two weeks. You can *do* this. It's a potluck and I will look after everything." Mike looked at me long and hard. "It'll take your mind off things for a bit. Don't you want that?"

I did want that. I *very much* wanted that. In fact, I wanted a giant whiteboard eraser that I could just wave in the air and erase this whole flippin' nightmare. I thought for several minutes, trying hard to hold my emotions in check. I drew in a long, deep breath and held it as I continued to think. I trusted Mike when he said we'd be okay, and with that trust came a bit of relief.

I let my breath out in a whoosh, my cheeks puffing a bit. "Okay." I nodded with conviction. "Let's do this."

When we'd purchased the house it had come fully furnished. Uniquely crafted wooden beds, great artwork and some cool nautical trinkets were definitely keepers, but old area rugs, dated curtains and a number of other items needed to go. We had our own belongings from our other homes as well and so we had our work cut out for us. Call us crazy, but we somehow managed to unpack forty-five boxes, assemble our twelve-foot-long farmhouse dining table (which weighs a ton and seats sixteen), make up beds, pull down curtains, roll up carpets, wash floors, and work our behinds off. Getting the house ready for our guests was a huge motivator and allowed us for a wee bit to forget about my shocking diagnosis.

That night, completely worn out, we lay down in bed and finally allowed the emotions to surface from the devastating news. Duey, our beloved English Mastiff, climbed up and gently parked himself between us. Mike and I continued to stare at each other, again, speechless. A heavy, vast sadness filled us and we were completely overcome with emotion. We cried; slowly and softly at first and then louder, fuller sobs took over. As we held each other, Duey started moaning long, mournful sounds. We could see that his eyes were watering. He knew something was very wrong, and he was equally devastated by our pain. As we hugged and cried, he stayed with us and eventually the three of us, completely broken hearted and physically drained, fell asleep. Duey, with his big, fuzzy head on my abdomen as always, quietly snored.

We had planned for our two adult girls, Annie and Maddie, to come over the next evening to see the new home. (We wanted them to see it first before the rest of the family were to come for brunch the morning after that.) Mike and I worked hard all that next day, and the girls and their partners arrived at five p.m., about thirty hours after we had received our mind-blowing news. *Would they know something was up?* I wondered, and tried my hardest to look cheery. These young women are hugely intuitive, and there is no hiding secrets or surprises. Somehow, miraculously, my diagnosis remained behind a tightly sealed vault, and we had a great night with a BBQ dinner, a few games of pool, and a late-night walk on the land.

Our realtor had shared a secret with us when we were initially looking at the property. "Rumour has it there is a very rare, old white deer who roams these parts. Because she is scarcely seen, one would be quite fortunate to come across her, so keep an eye out!" A white deer! Well. I promptly looked up white deer to learn that only one in about forty thousand exist. I highly doubted his story. Surely the rumour was fabricated to make the new property even more enchanting.

I hadn't shared this rumour with the girls, but we needed fresh air and it was decided that Annie and Maddie, along with their boyfriends, Duey, Mike, and I would all go for a nighttime walk. Outside, just feet from the ocean, was pitch-black—coastal life at its finest. We all crashed around and fumbled in the dark on our maiden evening voyage through forest. All of a sudden one of the guys yelled. "Holy shit! What *was* that? A ghost?" He sounded really scared.

Mike saw it too. "It's the white deer! Look!" The poor animal was startled and took off, breaking twigs and thumping the ground heavily as it bounded off. At first I was amazed to know it was here with us, but then I thought, *Of course it settled here. It too felt the amazing energy I felt on top of the hill.*

I was immensely relieved to have the distraction of the cheerful faces and laughter of the young adults visiting. My gosh, though, I felt like I was betraying them by acting like life was normal when inside I felt so upset. *And the academy award for best actress goes to . . . .* Each time I hugged them I felt very close to tears and I was exhausted by the effort it took not to break down. Later that night, as the kids were laughing and happy and so enthralled with this huge, beautiful log home of ours on the ocean, I almost forgot that I was sick. It was surreal to have these emotions, going back and forth.

The next morning was the housewarming brunch. It was a very jovial time as my parents, Mike's dad, Mike's sister, his aunt and her husband, the girls and their young men all gathered and celebrated with chilled mimosas, housewarming presents, and all the brunchy-food stuff you can imagine.

Just as we were about to eat, Mike's dad made an emotional toast. He outlined what a hellish year we'd had and how pleased he was that we had finally obtained this fine new home and that we were moving forward after all that we had been through. He told everyone how "impressed" he was by the strength we had as a couple "to get through so much." My heart pounded as I shot a sharp look at Mike: *Did you tell him?* my eyes asked. A slight head movement. No, he hadn't told him. It was just words.

Finally, brunch was finished, the crowd left, and Mike and I again were in a daze. We still hadn't really had any time to absorb the news, yet somehow we had managed to unpack and set up the house, have an evening with the kids, and host a brunch and house tour the following day. We collapsed on the bed, exhausted, and slept for the next five hours.

Monday we both went to work and acted like nothing had ever happened.

But before I go on, let's back up a bit.

4

DECIDUAL CAST

"**O**h my God!" I yelled. "What the hell?" It was April, seven months before the diagnosis. I was bleeding uncontrollably. Big globs of tissue were gushing out of me into the toilet. "What is happening?" It was as if a tap of blood was turned on and pouring out of me. I looked in the toilet. I called out to my husband, "I think I just birthed a bat!" A large, globby, red, clotty thing was in the toilet bowl. It indeed looked like a bat. I later learned this was a decidual or uterine cast, or better yet, a membranous dysmenorrhea. So, yeah, basically, a bat.

It was 11:30 p.m. We were flying to Ottawa at 7:30 a.m. the next morning to attend a getaway for my fifty-first birthday. We'd gone all-out with the plans to make up for missing my fiftieth—COVID had blown that birthday all to hell. I was excited to take in a country music concert. Chris Stapleton was my secret fantasy musician-lover, and I couldn't wait to celebrate with my hubby, my sister-in-law Janet, and our good friend Kyle. I came out of the bathroom exhausted and scared. "I think I need to head into Emergency."

I packed a bag with a few hospital things and we drove in to emerg. *Surely to God this is not what perimenopause is all about.* I had been an hour and a half sitting on the toilet with non-stop bleeding into the bowl. *How much blood had I lost?* Luckily I had packed for our Ottawa trip well in advance, as I was too excited to hold off. We hadn't had a vacation in a while. We ventured out into the dark, windy, rainy night on the twisty-turny highway. On nights like this, one should really be home, tucked snuggly in bed.

It was close to one o'clock when we arrived at the hospital. I was pale, frazzled, and blood-soaked completely down both legs. They took me in fairly quickly and ran the usual—blood work, blood pressure, an EKG— and asked an endless amount of questions about my habits, my lifestyle, and my health.

At about 2:00 am, Mike decided to drive home to get two or three hours of sleep and to grab our things for the trip. We realized I would not be going back to our house beforehand. We were hopeful we could still catch our early morning flight.

Another hour later, a doctor and a nurse came in and performed an internal exam. I was terrified they were going to say something was majorly wrong, especially with my nagging inner voice telling me I had cancer. "Well," the doc paused, "it looks pretty good in there!" I was quite relieved but also surprised. *Does this mean this is actually NORMAL?* The doc read my mind. "We will wait for the blood test results, but you know, probably nothing."

I sighed, and then thought, *They didn't do any imaging with CT, ultrasound, or X-ray. The human eye can't see inside the body. How can they be so sure I don't have cancer? I'm going to have to pursue this after my trip.* In hindsight, I'd have been so much further along in my treatment had they done their due diligence that night and run the diagnostics.

By 5:30 a.m. Mike was calling me and we were trying to assess if we would still make the flight to Ottawa. "We can do it!" I said with conviction. "Let's get to the concert!" Exhausted and stressed, I sucked it up and asked Mike to bring my suitcase and to pick me up at hospital. He high-tailed it out of the house and miraculously picked me up at 6:30. He is no wimp on the road and can handle himself at Mach speed quite comfortably. By seven o'clock we had picked up Kyle and then Janet and were racing to the airport. I was desperate for a shower, a little delirious from exhaustion and blood loss, and was trying hard to make the best of it.

Thankfully, it was a pretty uneventful flight. We landed in Ottawa and excitedly got settled into our hotel rooms. By dinnertime we had showered, eaten, enjoyed some drinks, and were ready for a night on the town. Kyle came into the room with a very long face. "Guys. You're not going to believe this. The Chris Stapleton concert is cancelled. One of the band members has COVID." In dis-belief, we stared at each other. Our hyped up, highly charged energy fell from up on the stucco ceiling right down to the spotted hotel carpet floor in about two seconds flat. We were all trying to keep our emotions in check, but we wanted to cry, yell, curse and even drown our sorrows . . . perhaps in a bottle of moonshine? We *loved* Chris Stapleton. Between the four of us we had dropped a few thousand dollars on flights, concert tickets, the hotel room, booze, food, and the rental car. I had marched on through my own fatigue, upset, physical pain and the worry of my unknown condition to make the trip. I had really needed this time to blow off steam, as we had had some very stressful years with moves, my ongoing health concerns, and of course, the perilous and still highly unknown age of COVID.

We decided to make the best of it and ended up basically playing cards and partying for two days straight. It was actually quite fun, but not how you want to spend time and money you hadn't planned on spending in place of a highly anticipated concert. We flew home, worn out and disappointed but having made the best of it. When we returned, I was surprised to see I had major fluid accumulation around my ankles. My legs were all puffed up. This was new.

I called my GP and told her about the events surrounding the emergency visit and what had happened. She met with me and reviewed the report. "Well, your liver enzyme markers are up and your FSH levels are high," she said casually. I asked what that meant and she shrugged it off. "Probably nothing." That was that. Probably nothing. Just regular symptoms. "You are at that age," she added.

Life went on. By June I had had more horrid bat birthing issues and daily, constant, heavy bleeding. The bleeding had now been going on for roughly eight months. "This isn't normal," I'd tell my family doctor. "I'm tired of all this. I don't feel right" The response back was always the same: "This is part of perimenopause. Get used to it."

I couldn't get used to it. I'd golf and be panting for breath. I'd walk the dog and feel like I needed to return home on a stretcher. My balance was off, my memory was bad, the night sweats were dreadful, and I had insomnia regularly. I know that a lot of these things are indeed perimenopause symptoms, but mine were beyond severe. And all the while, the nagging, intuitive voice was telling me I had cancer.

July came and I went back to the doc again. "Okay, this bleeding every day has been going on since October. I really feel something is *way* off. I mean c'mon, that's approaching nine months."

"Well," she said, "I can book you a biopsy, but you'll likely be through all of this by the time they see you. The wait for a biopsy is over a year. Why bother?"

We sat there, eye to eye. Her reasoning floored me. I explained I would rather her book it anyway in case I WAS still bleeding in a year's time.

So July sped into August and then September. The nagging voice inside my head was now basically yelling at me. I went to my doctor again. "Any way to call the biopsy place and see if I can get moved up?" I asked. I was so tired of all of this.

The doc sighed. "There's no way to get in sooner. Call them yourself if you like," she'd said it a little flippantly and then added, "see what you can find out."

So, I called. I explained how desperate I was and how awful my symptoms were. They said they would put me on a cancellation list, and, sure enough, I got in on October 24, only eight weeks later. I couldn't wait.

The day finally came for my appointment with the specialist. We discussed the symptoms and she said, "You know, some women go through this stuff just like you and it's nothing, all part of the perimenopause-al world." I stared at her. *Is she dismissing me? Trying to give me the brush off?* I was taught not to be rude or pushy, so had never been a self-advocate. There were five women in that small room with me: the specialist, two nurses, and two student observers. This had seemed like a lot of people to me, and I felt a bit out-numbered, but as the hospital's favourite saying goes, "This *is* a teaching hospital." *Screw it*, I thought. *I need to speak up.*

I looked at the specialist and pleaded. "Please. Please just do a biopsy." The specialist sighed. It was late in the day, and I think she just wanted to finish up and go home. Finally, she looked at me and said, "Okay, up you get. We may as well be sure." I climbed up on the table, she got herself organized, and the two nurses stood on either side of me as I laid down.

With my feet in position in the cold stirrups, the doctor pushed my knees open. She put on big, googly-eyed glasses that made her resemble a *Sesame Street* character. Then she put some sort of headlamp on, and for a second I thought she looked like a miner about to go exploring underground. I almost said this to make light of the situation. After a few minutes of investigating, she said loudly, "Good God, woman, do you always have all this brown gunky stuff in here?" I couldn't believe she had made this thoughtless and crude comment at all, let alone in front of the other four women. I was stunned at her lack of professionalism. I thought to myself, *"Well, lady, how would I know? It's kinda hard to get my eyeballs down between my legs to look back up inside myself. I'm not an ostrich!"* I wished I had had the courage to say it out loud. The room was quiet. I said nothing but nervously shrugged. I had told her at this point that I had been bleeding non-stop for close to a year, so I'm not sure what she was expecting, but I wasn't at all surprised by the "miner's" discoveries. Knowing now what I hadn't known then, I'm pretty sure she was seeing the cancer. Her comment, and my thoughts of contorting myself like an ostrich, brought back some vivid childhood memories of travelling in the family car during the holidays. I think I was about eight years old at the time . . .

We were making the long journey to Saint John, New Brunswick to visit our Nana. We usually made the trek during the March Break while my sister and I had a week off from school. Back in the 70's, the month of March in the Maritimes was quite snowy and, as usual, the five-hour car ride turned into about seven hours, due to icy roads and overly cautious drivers.

Because I possessed not-yet-diagnosed ADHD, and, because I was experiencing a severe case of the fidgets, I was unable to sit still any longer in the back seat of the family car. I started singing, squirming, telling jokes and dancing. I tried to entertain myself as best I could all the while wearing my seatbelt. Unfortunately, those lap-belts could get awfully tight when one squirmed around and I really wanted to just un-buckle it to get my Saturday Night Fever moves perfected. Of course, Mom was adamant that the seatbelts were to remain fastened and, even with all of my extra efforts with well-planned car toys, I was ready to spontaneously combust.

My sister, who was desperately trying to sleep the time away, was getting annoyed. "Mom" she complained, "Andrea is bugging me! Make her stop!" Flabbergasted, I turned and looked at her with my mouth agape; I could not believe my ears. I'd been doing my very best to entertain myself. I'd already read a Hardy Boys book, colored two horses and a barn, completed several word finds and a crossword puzzle, and even attempted to knit a Lopi sweater. With all the fidgeting, my crackers and snacks had gotten all crumbly and caught up in the yarn, so I'd packed that up neatly in my sock. I'd played and broken my Rubik's cube, jammed my plastic party favor and, even with the extraordinary amount of effort trying to entertain myself, had ultimately started with the fidgets.

No one in those days understood why I had such excess energy. Truly, I had done my absolute best to get this far in the car. As a child, I had visions of someday being an actress on stage. And so, in my best Southern-belle accent, I feigned shock and loudly protested. "Lara! You're a liar!" Proclaiming the truth, I'd yelled those words with all my might. I heard audible gasps. (I was prepared to win accolades over this loud announcement.) "Stop it Andrea! Right now! You're this close to being grounded again!" Mom yelled. I sat there for a moment, trying to figure out what had just happened. I looked at my sister. *How was I bugging her? Had I looked at her the wrong way? Had I bumped her?* I examined the cooler in between us. It was still exactly in the middle. My checklist was clear; I'd done nothing wrong.

I sat there for a minute thinking about what my mom had said; or yelled rather. *What was it that I should stop doing?* I really had no clue. I resumed my head shaking; pushing my hands on the seat to bounce my skull around extra fast. I put my hands over my ears and pulled them off quickly and repeatedly to make the cool vacuum noise that the compressed air made. I opened my window and put my long hair out to make it fly wildly around in twisty circles. I made my teddy bear dance, practicing his Rockette moves; and I proudly observed that he was getting pretty good. I practiced weird noises; armpit farts, snorts, and fake giggles -for when I really needed them. "She's doing it again!" Lara protested. I looked over at her. "What??" I asked. I had been so careful not to bother her. What I hadn't understood however, was that my *actions* were what was bugging her.

My dad looked at my mother. "Do I need to pull the car over?" he asked quietly. I was horrified. "Dad! Why would you need to pull the car over? What's wrong with the car? Do we have a flat tire? Are we out of gas? Is a moose chasing us?" Now this last thought really cracked me up. The first two were legit questions on my part. I hadn't put two and two together that he was asking in case he had to deal with *me*. I sat there smiling as I thought the moose comment was really quite funny. In my mind I could picture this giant moose, bug eyed, racing against the car, snow flying everywhere, the swingy, furry thing under his chin bobbing back and forth . . . *what was that thing called anyway?* My mind wandered and I laughed out loud. Unfortunately, my parents were both saying important things to me during this time and I had missed all of it. The timing of my laughter coincided with them telling me I was being saucy. *I* didn't know I was being saucy.

Maybe it was the stress of being on a wintery highway, or maybe Mom was just really tired; she lost all of her patience with me. "Ok Andrea Leigh! You're behaving like a real . . . shit-head!" she exploded in sheer frustration. I sensed, finally, that the three of them were really annoyed with me. I desperately tried to lighten the mood. "Hmmmm." I wondered out loud, arms crossed and my index finger tapping on my chin. "What exactly *is* a shit head?" A smirk crossed my face. I knew I was really pushing my luck; this was a bad word coming out of my mouth right in front of my parents. My dad huffed. My sister turned full on to stare at me with a wide open mouth and huge eyes. My mother officially lost it. In a very loud voice she yelled, "Well Andrea, bend over and stick your head up your ass, and you'll find out!!" Complete silence. The words stuffed in the over-packed car were simply hanging in waiting. No one knew what to say or do for a good five seconds. Dad made some odd, disgusted sound, and clacked his tongue.

Lara yelled "Mom!" in absolute horror, and Mom? well she just laughed like a madwoman and cried at the same time. My mind, however, was already off to the races, as I sat there trying to figure out if somehow, with my bendy gymnastic body, I could actually stick my head up my ass.

I'm not really sure how long I'd laid there with this family flash back playing, but when I came back to reality, the gynecologist had the items ready to perform the biopsy, and the nurses had put their hands on my stomach. Sternly, they instructed, "This is going to hurt. Don't lift your bum or arch your back or it'll make things feel a lot worse." All of a sudden I felt a hot, searing rip, deep in my insides. "Argh!" I yelled and sucked in air. I screwed up my face, winced in pain, and scrunched my toes. I know I squeezed the heck out of somebody's hand. "Oh my God!" I cried out, through clenched teeth. I breathed in deeply and felt tears spring to my eyes as the two women firmly held me down. The pain was severe; it took my breath away and lasted several minutes. Clearly the nurses were used to this reaction and calmly said, "Breathe. Just breathe." They tried to look reassuring.

"Okay, missus." The doc nodded, all casual. "Probably nothing. We will call ya in about two weeks."

5

THE EAGLE

In some cultures, the eagle is a powerful representation of all things ethereal, a messenger from the highest gods. Having grown up in a small town just outside of a busy city, I didn't have any experience, knowledge or opinion regarding eagles. In elementary school we'd learned that their wingspan can be as wide as eight feet, the female is larger than the male, and that they are the emblem of many countries. I knew they were revered, and I knew it was likely game over for most things that an eagle spies to eat, but I had absolutely no idea that a vast number of people in various parts of our world associate the eagle with spiritual messaging.

A year prior to my diagnosis, my mother had been scheduled for spinal surgery at the ripe old age of eighty. I was quite nervous for her. Each time she ever has a surgery—eyes, knees, you name it—it gets botched. A hole poked through a retina, a clot in the knee—what should all go perfectly smoothly, never does. It gets messy and complicated, every single time. When she realized she would need a person with her, I dutifully committed. And so, on this particular morning, I dropped her off and naturally had a really bad feeling for her. "Goodbye, Mom." I hugged her. "You'll do fine!" We hugged a little too long as we nervously and silently wondered if she could withstand another general anesthetic. Her heart wasn't great. A nervous smile and a "See you when you wake up!" and I was outta there.

I picked up Duey and brought him to our regular park, which was always very quiet. I only ever see maybe one other dog off-leash whenever I'm there. When you have a reactive, two-hundred-pound guard dog, a quiet park like this hidden gem is golden. I unclipped the leash to release him and he took off, sniffing away, tail wagging. I marvelled at the day—a clear blue sky, crisp air, the familiar sounds and smells of the nearby harbour. I felt blessed and full of gratitude. I decided to say a little prayer for Mom . . . it couldn't hurt. I closed my eyes and stood still. I prayed, *"Creator of our universe, please be with my mother on this journey. Please allow her surgery to be a success and watch over her as best you can. I will be eternally grateful. Amen."*

I stood there for a moment with my eyes closed, imagining the surgery and picturing everything. Suddenly I heard a swishing sound and opened my eyes. To my amazement, right in front of me was a gigantic bald eagle, sitting on the grass. Staring straight at me, it turned its head quizzically. Noting its piercing gaze, I was both nervous and amazed. I glanced at Duey. He was oblivious. I sighed some relief. The last thing I needed was a horrific battle between a giant, powerful, wild bird with a sharp beak, razor talons, and the wingspan of a small bus, and a four-legged, heavy-weight, hairy, drooling, toothy beast whose jaws were more powerful than almost all land animals and who possessed a natural, pack-like instinct to protect me at all costs. I was afraid just thinking about it, although it would be an impressive fight.

I continued to stare at the bird. *"Your mother will be fine, Andrea. We are with her."* The voice in my head surprised me. *Was that a message from the eagle?* Very carefully I walked toward it while simultaneously reaching for my phone. Incredibly, it continued to just quietly sit there, watching me. I snapped a few photos and then my phone rang. I jumped. I had not been aware of the adrenalin coursing through my veins. It was the hospital calling. Mom was fine and they were confident the surgery had been a success. I cried tears of relief and voiced my thanks to the staff. I hung up and loudly exclaimed, "Thank you, Lord!" Smiling, I turned back to look at the eagle, but it was gone.

6

KISMET

When Mike and I got married, the wedding was held on his family's private, oceanfront property in beautiful, rural Nova Scotia. It was an outdoor wedding with 120 guests, all gathered under a giant, white tent. It was fall . . . and it made for an exceptionally beautiful setting. Because we loved the property so very much, we also dreamt of someday building our forever home on this same piece of land

Annie and Maddie were eleven and nine years old at the time of the wedding, and, like me, they too walked down the aisle in ivory dresses, silver and pearl head bands and carried an array of flowers. Smiling, youthful and so very beautiful, they resembled little princesses and took our breath away. Mike was not only marrying me, but was also officially becoming their step-dad.

For the time being, we were living in my family home, knowing full well that our time there would eventually come to an end. We'd planned to pack up and begin the long journey toward building our forever home once the girls had graduated from high school.

My family home held two generations of memories. I'd lived there from age four and had grown up in the house with Lara and my parents. After several wild and adventurous years away in my early twenties, I eventually moved back home and purchased the house from my father, ready to raise my own two daughters from infancy to young adulthood under that very same roof.

Time has its own way of quietly passing on, and in the blink of an eye, both girls had graduated from high school and we were ready to list. I had worked hard at making the house thoroughly appealing; every room free of clutter and with a warm, cozy vibe. Not surprisingly, it sold quickly.

Closing day came, and as everyone who has ever sold a family home truly knows, the feelings on that day were bittersweet. I looked around at the empty rooms and gleaming floors, and I said one last, emotional goodbye. I reassured myself that our plans were for the best. Our street had become very traffic-laden, not the right spot for future grandchildren. Still, it stung a bit. Our house was in a lovely area and we had fantastic neighbours, some of whom were our very best friends.

As I walked through the house one last time, going from room to room and saying goodbye, flashbacks of years past whizzed through my mind. So many memories. I stood in the entryway remembering the kids when they were little, watching them carefully tying their sneakers as I waited to walk them to school; giggling and playing out front on the old tire swing; exploring the backyard with Easter egg hunts; climbing the giant rock walls; eating popcorn in the living room; having sleepovers; doing the limbo in the kitchen during New Year's Eve parties. And the Christmases, oh how I'd loved those. We'd had the biggest Christmases with the biggest Christmas trees. There were baby christenings, birthday parties, graduations, and guitar jams . . . . with all of those memories, selling our house was a big deal.

We had purchased two downtown condos in the early stages of construction in the hopes of flipping them in two years' time to put money toward our dream home. We figured this was a good plan and thought the location would be fun for a few years while we sorted ourselves out. We hoped to enjoy concerts, restaurants, hockey games, and walks along the waterfront. But we were in a small unit and soon became quite miserable. From our condo, motorcycles, ambulances, and late-night partiers could be heard all night long on the street below, and the wall between our den and the neighbour's bedroom was embarrassingly thin, making it awkward each time we ran into them.

Walking our beloved Duey downtown was an absolute nightmare.

Because of his sheer size and handsomeness, strangers couldn't seem to walk by without reaching out to pat him on the head; he was a novel attraction to say the least. Sadly, for a guard dog, those random strangers at unexpected times stressed him out and he was always in a heightened state, jumping up or mouthing people he didn't know. He would bark and lunge at scooters and skateboarders, and his overly protective nature ended up becoming problematic. He became known to the locals as the "giant, rearing horse," dragging us all over the streets and chasing down "threats." And then, brutally, only a few months after we moved into the new building, the COVID-19 pandemic hit. We were basically trapped inside a tiny Kleenex box with our 200-pound beast and nowhere to go. This spurred me on to begin quickly designing our dream home.

I painstakingly learned how to create and lay out the house plans on our computer, only to have them disappear twice—once from a glitch in the free app, and a second time because the online company just disappeared. Uncountable hours lost, I got out the graph paper and then designed it old-school.

After many tedious hours of erasing, rulers, and research, I created a three-floor, six-thousand-square-foot home on five pieces of graph paper all carefully taped together. It was an incredible floor plan, and I readily admit, I was obsessed with the project. I had a giant binder full of rooms, each one carefully planned and measured out exactly. I had fabric samples, paint chips, and furniture layouts. I proudly showed all of our friends the architectural designs; they were in awe at the amount of work, the creativity, and the scope of what I'd detailed. Many people told me I had the potential to become both an interior designer and an architect.

With the plans officially entered into Mike's computer software, we hired a construction company and their architect also loved our design. Soon it was placed on the company website, and clients told them it was the best design yet! I chuckled, as it was created by *me*, not their designers. My feathers were fluffed.

Before long we found ourselves picking out flooring, lighting, and appliances, and we met on the property to stake out the land. We were truly very happy and excited to have finally arrived to this point. Our dreams were coming true, and soon we would have our dream home, our . . . *forever* home. As we got closer to breaking ground for the beginning of the build, I finally again envisioned dinner parties, fancy Christmases, grandchildren, guitar parties, mastiff puppies (lots!) running around, and I looked forward to an amazing space to spend our days. Mike had committed countless hours over the past two years orchestrating the selling of the house and both condo units and managing all of the paperwork and lawyer meetings and was very glad that it was all finally coming to an end.

By this point we were living in the basement at the family cottage on the land we were married and where we were to build. One day I came home and unexpectedly met Mike in the driveway. He looked awful. "Mike?" I asked, as I quickly got out of the car, "What's happened?" He walked over to me and collapsed into my arms, deeply sighing. "It's the house. Our permit was denied and we can't build. Our future here is not even possible." And just like that, our dreams had been snuffed out like a candle flame.

I was stunned. *What on earth?* The news devastated us as we had met our plans head-on with much thoroughness and tremendous effort. My mind raced as I replayed the exhausting and very stressful past two years; the efforts to pack up, sell and move two generations worth of belongings from our family home, the move into and then sale of the larger condo after only nineteen months and then the additional move with all of our belongings to the smaller condo. Three months after moving to the smaller condo, we sold that one as well and again packed everything up. After a long twenty-two months of stress, frustration, and worry, (the units were structural nightmares and lawsuits waiting to happen) we were relieved to finally move on but we then were left essentially homeless as the buyers' closing date was earlier than we'd hoped and we had nothing lined up to move into.

We looked for short-term rentals but quickly learned that no one wanted to rent a space to a couple with a mastiff. Apparently, some people can't even acquire house insurance with that breed of dog. With no options available, we had to move to our little winter ski cottage, ninety minutes from the city. Mike commuted back and forth a fair amount during the span of a month while we waited to relocate to Mike's family cottage at the end of the summer.

Once we got settled into the family cottage, we made the tough decision to pack up our winter property to put on the market as well. Oh how we'd loved that place. We designed it ourselves and had spent a great deal of time there, but we were fuelled by the end goal of pooling all of the money from sales and building the dream home we had envisioned for so long.

And so, having moved to the basement of Mike's family cottage with a life's worth of items all packed into storage, it seemed we were just inches away from the final steps in the overall plans. All of this chaos and a total of four moves had happened within an exhausting two-year time frame, and we had faced much conflict in the trials and tribulations of purchasing, selling, packing, and moving, repeat, repeat, repeat. We rallied with the sole focus of building and settling on the land on which we were married. The "happily ever after" was worth the constant packing and unpacking, the time spent adjusting to each new space, and the preparation of properties to get them "show ready," but we were quickly running out of steam and just barely holding on for the end goal.

"I can't believe this has happened." Mike's voice brought me back to the present. Looking at his face sent me reeling. I suddenly felt exasperated and very angry.

"What do you mean? Why can't we build?" Yelling now, I started to panic. I was aware of how I sounded but just couldn't help it; I was shocked and bitterly disappointed. He explained that unbeknownst to any of us, there was a municipal bylaw that states you must have 100-foot frontage on a public road. Our spacious property was on a private lane and only accessible *through* that lane. We couldn't expand it as houses existed on either side before our property line started. Therefore, we had zero frontage. This apparently would pose issues for emergency vehicles etc. The bylaw was only uncovered when the application for the permit was submitted.

This unexpected news destroyed us. It was a double whammy—we were left with no future plans and once again had no place to go. We'd sold every property we owned and now felt completely lost.

We decided to pursue the permit issue. We met with lawyers, town planners, politicians, and after about six months of hopes repeatedly crushed, finally threw in the towel.

"What now?" I asked. I did not want to move back to the city.

Mike took a deep breath. "Well, we look at our options and start to search for property."

And so began another six months of house hunting and raw emotions. We remained discouraged and exhausted.

One day, Mike texted me a real estate link to a beautiful house. It was on the ocean and just six minutes away from his family property. He was in New York. "Check it out!" he said. I wasn't really expecting much; this was the twelfth house we'd looked at. We had seen beautiful, expensive properties that just didn't do it for me. They didn't have that magic *feel* of a home. I wanted the place to have a feel. I didn't care if the driveway was newly paved or there were five bedrooms or a brand-new kitchen—I'd live in a cave if it felt right energetically. So I drove over by myself with pretty low expectations.

As I came to the address and turned up the long driveway, I recall exclaiming, "Ooh, this *is* nice!" The driveway wound around big trees and boulders and brought me into a private, nestled world. I saw several adult deer quietly grazing in a field, and as I came to the top of the hill, the view of the ocean was just below. This intrigued me. I slowly drove down into the parking area. My body reacted; the hairs on my arms stood on end. "What is going on?" I whispered. I marvelled at the tingles in my body. I got out of the car. *Welcome home, Andrea,* my inner voice said. But really, *was* it my inner voice? Or was something else out there in the universe saying welcome home *to* me, in my head, guiding me to be here. Do you ever wonder about that? Our subliminal thoughts? Who's really sending them? *What is that all about?* I wondered again, *Am I saying "Welcome home" to myself because somehow, without even seeing inside, I know intrinsically that this is the right place to be?* I chuckled at the thought.

The realtor had not yet arrived, and I debated whether I should explore a bit or wait in my car. Several minutes passed and I couldn't resist a second longer. Heart pounding, I got out of the car, closed the door behind me and took in the incredible scenery. A huge log home with mature gardens, immaculate lawns, and the sounds of the beautiful, rolling ocean brought me unexpected joy. I felt a huge smile cross my face.

Behind the house to my right was a short, sandy path to the beach, and I walked down the hill toward the ocean. I admired again the tranquility of it all. The surf was gently bubbling up on the shore and instantly it comforted me. I've always felt that there's something deeply cleansing about waves, and on this day I was full of gratitude for being in the ocean's presence.

It felt like I was on a cultivated movie set. It was . . . perfect. I looked back up the hill to a smiling man. "Hi, Andrea!" He waved. "Wanna go inside?"

At the time, I didn't know I had cancer, and I was embarrassed at how out of breath I was walking back up the hill. The realtor opened the door for me, and the inside of this beautiful home took my breath away. Logs no less than eighteen inches thick, and floor to ceiling windows. From these windows, the ocean looked just an arm's reach away. Three floors, all open concept, two guest bedrooms for the girls—it was a dream space to be sure. I was stunned. I felt instantly at home and stayed there for an hour. "I'm sorry," I said to the realtor, "I just don't want to leave this space!"

He laughed. "Well, my dear, that is a sure sign that the house is yours!"

I took the papers on the property from the realtor and regretfully drove away. I felt torn to leave, even on that very first day. Never in my life had I felt this strongly grounded about anywhere I'd lived, and I've lived in over a dozen places between houses, apartments, condos, and university residences.

I called Mike in New York. "You have to see this place!" He was coming home in two days. "Can I book another showing?" I begged.

"Sure," he said, but I heard the caution in his voice. He could tell I was in love with the space, and he was worried he'd be the one who would have to break my heart.

After the call, I walked down to the family dock with Duey. We'd gone down there every day for the past year. Since selling the condos, we were camped out in the lower level of the family cottage and our afternoon habit was dockside. I sat in a chair and listened to the cove water gently lapping against the dock—such a lovely spot. I decided to pray. I rarely pray for myself, but today, I prayed with all my heart: *"Dear Creator, divine master of all things in our universe, please hear my prayer and guide me along the right path. I have found a home. I feel like this is the right space for us. I know Mike is worried about this decision. If this indeed is the path for us, perhaps allow us to somehow know this and to have the confidence to move ahead. Amen."*

I nodded to myself, as if to seal the deal. Out of nowhere, a huge, powerful eagle with a giant wingspan circled overhead. Never in the year of daily dock visits had I witnessed this majestic creature. It stayed, flying around me for quite some time. "Oh my God!" I exclaimed through my tears, remembering back to my mother's operation a year earlier, and the eagle that had visited me in the park that day only moments after I'd prayed. "There's the sign!"

Shortly after that, Mike came home from New York. The next day we drove over together to view the property. Again my mind raced. *Will I feel the same way I did the other day? With fresh eyes, will I still see things in the same vein?* We got out of the car and my heart started to pound. I tried hard not to show my exuberance as I didn't want to put any pressure on Mike. We walked the property and went inside. I could tell he loved it; he is a softie for a good log home. He asked all the usual questions—information about the well, the septic system, how it was heated, age of the roof, blah, blah, blah. I was nervous. *What if there is something we missed?*

After a long time, we drove back to the family property. We had a lot to consider. We both knew what this decision would mean. If we went ahead with the purchase, the hopes and dreams of living in our forever home on the family's secluded, expansive, country property would revert back to just that—a dream. Hopes were now dashed that our future would come to fruition in the home I had so painstakingly designed for the land on which we were married. With no hope for an immediate resolution to the bylaw, we had to consider the impacts of purchasing another property and putting our plans on the back burner. It was a big decision for Mike, and I could tell he was torn.

I went down the large hill to the dock at the cove, to clear my head. After a while I called him on his cell. "C'mon down with some drinks and let's try to sort through this." Hopeful, I hung up. He came down a while later and was visibly stressed. He was concerned about giving up the exhaustive efforts regarding the bylaw for the build. Our future looked obscure and uncertain; if we chose to continue living in the family cottage waiting for the bylaw to be reversed, it could take years.

I decided to pray again. I asked that the Creator guide us. I asked that Mike gain the ability to see his way through this by making a decision that was best for him, and for us, for once to put his own needs first. We had to accept that our dreams of living on the family land were not possible. We had pursued and fought it long enough. It was time to let go.

Exhausted, I finished my prayer. I sat quietly. It felt good to turn this over to a higher power. We sat there together, quietly, for a short while when suddenly, Mike exclaimed, "Well there's something you don't see every day!" He was pointing to the sky. I looked in the direction in which he was pointing. To my amazement, quietly flying over us, not one, but TWO eagles circled overhead.

7

MOVING WEEK

I very much believe in divine intervention. Ultimately, my prayers were answered, and with great joy we purchased the log home. And, like all the other moves before it, I packed diligently, efficiently, and quickly. I noticed that this time though, I was truly exhausted. "I don't want to do this anymore," I lamented. "I am so sick of packing and unpacking." This was now our fifth complete move in a three-year span, and I was feeling deeply, profoundly tired. It was quite obvious that things were not right but I couldn't understand the huge fatigue. As I walked boxes to the car, I kept stopping. My heart pounded, I was out of breath and felt like I needed to go to bed.

"You can do it! Just a few more boxes," Mike said.

"Nope," I said, a finality to my voice, "I am done."

Now, I'm a Taurus, and we are known for our stubbornness. I give my all, and then I give some more. And after that, when I'm about to keel over from sheer exhaustion, I still try to squeeze out just a little bit more. And then, still not ready to give up, I push out the last drop of energy I possibly have. So, when I get to the point of saying, "I'm done," I am DONE. Like, done-done. Not a remote, mouse-sized, miniscule bit of energy left to add. Mike knew what I meant.

It was Monday afternoon. We were trying to finish packing up boxes, because the movers were coming the next day. Even as excited as we were, I just couldn't bring myself to carry out another one. It was a lovely, cool day in October and yet I was so wiped that by four-thirty I staggered to the car and promptly fell asleep, my face wedged between the window and the seatbelt. I can't recall feeling that completely spent in all of my fifty-one years.

We made our way over to the new house that evening, and I assessed what was still left to do to direct the movers with the impending hundreds of boxes coming in just a few short hours. The pressure of being ready for their arrival was completely overwhelming, and it left me feeling uncharacteristically drained. "Hey, Mike?" I called, as he slogged a few of our most precious heavy boxes from the overly stuffed van, trying to get ahead of the game, "You should probably know that I don't really have a plan yet for what goes where." Not only did I need to plan where our own things were going, but suddenly was also tasked with planning for how to navigate around all of the existing furniture as well. We'd purchased the house fully furnished.

He looked at me in surprise. "Well that's not like you!" He looked at me a minute longer and then came over to my side. Typically, I would be racing around on adrenalin, a drink in one hand and a clipboard in the other, totally in control, organized, and with energy to spare.

"You know what? I'm just going to deal with all of this tomorrow. I'm really wiped." I was actually feeling disappointed and confused by my lack of stamina. "I'm too old for this!" I quipped, as I plodded off to a couch. And so I slumbered deeply, my body fighting diligently to rejuvenate.

Moving day went well with the movers, and everyone worked exceptionally hard. Even though there were six of us, after a short while, I again began staggering around. Mike brought over a chair, took me by the hand, and told me to sit down outside by the front door. "Just direct the movers where to go—up, down, top floor, et cetera," he said, eternally my fixer. I felt embarrassed sitting in the chair, as I wanted to be unpacking boxes and processing things too. I could not figure out why I was feeling just so terrible.

Fast-forward three days, and sadly, we knew the answer.

8
MOM'S THE WORD

After our gruelling week unpacking a huge house-load of boxes, the devastating cancer diagnosis, the weekend with the kids, and hosting the brunch, Monday morning arrived all too quickly. It hit HARD. VERY hard. Mike and I drove into the city to work. I was teaching guitar classes and going from client to client in a distracted daze. I was crying on the inside while outwardly I was smiling, singing, playing my guitar, and bipping around like life was one big party. "Congratulations on the new house!" everyone would say. "You must be sooo happy!" "You have the perfect life!" I would smile at them and nod and was left feeling like I was either an imposter or horribly ungrateful. I struggled to feel the joy or to comment much at all.

I managed to keep the façade up for about a week and a half, and ultimately called the oncologist. "Uh, how do I get through this? Should I be working?"

"No!" She was surprised. "You absolutely should not be working. You need to rest." Well, this was good news. Now all I had to do was unpack the rest of my house, plan for Annie's birthday, host a dinner party for eight friends, play through a series of song sets at my guitar party with fourteen women, organize a Christmas tree decorating event, host Christmas Eve, Christmas Day, and New Year's. Easy-peasy.

"So, when will my hysterectomy be?" I asked hesitantly, hoping somehow it would magically fall in between all that I had planned.

"Somewhere in the next six weeks," she replied. *Okay, perfect*, I foolishly thought. *By January I will be on my way to healing and feeling better.*

I told Mike I needed to take time off, and we discussed when we should tell the girls. I knew this would be devastating news—so very upsetting and worrisome for them both. Annie had a birthday coming up, and after that, Maddie had university exams. I didn't want to wreck either of those things with the worry and distraction that would ensue after they learned the news. Then I realized we would be into Christmas; I wasn't about to ruin *that* for the entire family, so, inevitably, we chose to keep it a secret.

There was, however, a small problem. My mother. She, amongst a list of other accomplishments in her lifetime of varied careers, had been an obstetrics nurse. She saw my fluid-filled belly in the summer and also knew of all of my health issues from the past year. She had pushed to hear more on my biopsy results. Each and every day from mid-October onward, she'd called and asked, "Did you get your results yet? When is your biopsy due back?"

I dodged the questions and nervously fibbed each time. "Not yet."

She was baffled. She kept saying, "This is rather odd. It shouldn't take this long." And I would agree and act like nothing was wrong. It bothered me greatly to have to do this, but I had no choice. I couldn't tell her and then risk the girls finding out when I felt so strongly about protecting them.

Late in November I woke suddenly in the middle of the night. While I was up, I checked my phone. To my surprise, I saw a text from Mom. She had called an ambulance and was headed to the hospital. I was shocked to read this and glanced at the time that it had been sent: 1:00 a.m. I glanced at the time now: 2:30. I called her. She answered on the first ring. She was crying and in tremendous pain. She was crying so hard in fact, she could barely speak, and this was very disturbing to me. Mom is tough, a legend even. She never cries. My older daughter, Annie, once said, "Mom, Nana is so tough! One time she dropped a heavy knife and the tip landed straight in her foot and she just pulled it out and kept making a salad!" That moment left a lasting impression on all of us, and to this day, we still think she is invincible.

You can imagine my concern when I heard her crying. "What's going on?" I asked.

"Oh, hi, dear," she said, sounding horrible. "I'm okay, but I've called an ambulance because the darn discs in my back are in spasm and I've been standing for the past hour and a half in the kitchen because I can't sit down. I am exhausted and in agony and I just wanted to let you know that I was going to the hospital. I texted you in hopes you would read my message in the morning and know what was happening. I'm sorry if I woke you."

The Nova Scotia medical system is an absolute mess. There is a shortage of both family doctors and specialists. The wait time for an appointment with a family doctor is typically about three weeks, and yet many people have no doctor at all. People who have the need for medical assistance then end up at emerg even if it's not a true emergency because clinics are filled up and the wait list for a family GP is extensive. Because of the sheer volume of people in emerg, the wait times in there can be as long as twenty-four hours. People have in fact died in the waiting room. For those with a true emergency, such as a bacterial infection, a broken femur, slipped discs, etc., that kind of wait is a painful hell and often times extremely dangerous. So, in the more severe cases, people have started calling ambulances to take them to the hospital. That way, there is a faster assessment, medical help, and the paramedics are obligated to stay with you while you lie on a stretcher until an emerg doctor can see you. At least paramedics can provide pain medication. Unfortunately, this causes an ambulance shortage, and it can take up to three hours or more for an ambulance to arrive. I was worried Mom would be waiting a lot longer than she thought.

Mom, however, was quite confident the paramedics would be there soon, but I did not like the way she sounded. "I'm on my way," I said.

"No, Andrea, I don't want you driving in. It's dark and storming out, and it's the middle of the night." Indeed, it was. And I was exhausted and dealing with my cancer diagnosis silently and therefore not getting much sleep. Truthfully, though, these situations fall on me, because my sister lives in California and Mom lives alone. I hung up and immediately walked out the door into the wind and the cold rain, still in my pajamas. I drove as fast as I could; the forty-five-minute drive done in thirty. *Andrea Andretti wins again!*

I arrived to Mom's in the dark of night and saw no ambulance and no paramedics. *Ridiculous.* I rushed in to find just Mom, alone, sweating and barely able to speak as she was in so much pain and fighting exhaustion. "Oh my gosh, Mom, why are you still standing?"

She looked at me, pale, lips pressed hard together, trying to cope. "I can't sit, Andrea. I've been holding on to this table for two hours. My legs are trembling and ready to give out, but my spine is in horrific spasm and I am afraid my discs will crumble. It could paralyze me."

I assessed the situation and decided that if she actually collapsed we might have even bigger problems—a concussion, a broken bone . . . . I hastily brought a chair over and told her she was going to sit down with my help. I showed her how to keep her back as straight as she could, just like she had been doing while standing, and I instructed, "Bend carefully at the knees and lower yourself. You can do this." She was terrified. Her back pain was out of control. After several minutes of coaxing and assisting, deep breaths and cries, we did it. I got her positioned.

We stayed like that for another hour. Imagine if I hadn't come when I did! I was worried for her and outwardly trying to support her, while inwardly feeling scared, sad, and desperately needing the comfort of my mother. I almost told her my cancer news right then and there, but with the strength of a soldier, I kept my secret. I so wanted the comfort she could give me, but I chose silence. So there we sat, in the quiet hours of the night, both of us exhausted. Eventually the ambulance came and she was taken to the hospital. I made the long drive home again and arrived just as the sun was coming up.

Another few weeks went by, and I ultimately decided that I would tell my family that I needed a full hysterectomy. I figured this would buy me some time and would explain the biopsy results by simply saying I was told I needed a hysterectomy and that that was all I knew. Well. My mother was again suspicious and said that that information was very odd. She continued to grill me. I miraculously maintained my silence and hosted Annie's birthday, a tree decorating party, potlucks, the guitar party, Christmas Eve, and an epic Christmas Day complete with a full turkey dinner. All of these moments passed by while I remained in a surreal, greatly worried, heavily distracted state. I smiled through it all like life was normal, while on the inside I was more than desperate to share our news. I needed family support and the effort it took to wait this out took its toll on me.

9
BREAKING THE NEWS

January finally arrived and I faced the fact that I desperately needed to communicate what was going on. I still hadn't been given the surgery date even though back in the first week of November I was told it would be within six weeks. *Good ol' Nova Scotia health care.* I wanted to tell Annie and Maddie first, as I absolutely could not risk them finding out through someone else. I knew that once Mom knew, it would be tricky for others to be around her without her spilling the beans; of course, like any mother, when it comes to these sorts of things, she doesn't really have a poker face.

The girls' schedules kept misaligning. Finally, one day, I nervously said, "Look, I need you both to come out so we can discuss the logistics of my hysterectomy." I felt absolutely sick about telling them. Years ago, I had to tell them that their father and I were getting a divorce. That day just about destroyed me, seeing their sweet cherub faces forever changed. And, up until this moment, that horrible day was truly the hardest thing I'd ever had to do. And now, once more, I had to share some utterly devastating news. Knowing the impact it was going to have on them made it just so unthinkably awful. It would break their hearts. I spent many sleepless nights thinking about how to tell them, and I went through endless tissues wiping away tears and blowing my nose. I had to remind myself to breathe deeply and to really focus all of my strength on controlling my huge emotions when the time came.

Finally, I was able to get them in the same place. They walked in, full of smiles and funny stories that would usually fill me up. I immediately felt my emotions rise up, and I fought hard not to cry on the spot. My body started to tremble, and I walked quickly around to the kitchen to busy myself so they wouldn't see the effort it took to keep myself in check. I felt like my ears were buzzing as my heart thumped heavily in my chest. I concentrated on their voices, their laughter, and started to relax a little, looking at their sweet faces and listening to them talk. They are such a joy, we are all very close and I am truly at my happiest when our little family circle of four is all together in our home.

We drank tea and had a snack of some sort, and all the while my mind raced and my heart continued to pound. It took everything I had not to just blurt it out and to break down crying. A mother often experiences such a twisted role; I had devastating news of my own health, feeling terrified and needing to be comforted, yet still trying to be their protector, to reassure them, to hold them and to keep their hearts intact.

We were laughing at something when, out of the blue, Maddie asked me what the status was on the hysterectomy, my biopsy, and how I was feeling. I was drying the dishes, trying to keep busy. *There's your cue*, I thought, feeling even more dread. I took a deep breath, walked slowly over to them, and sat. I explained it as carefully as I could. "Well, as you know, I have to get a hysterectomy, so that I can stop the miserable bleeding I experience every day. What you don't know is that they actually found a bit of cancer in there." Boom. It was out. *Finally*. I held my breath. I watched as their sweet faces went white. They both swallowed hard and tried to remain in control, but I could see their energy shift and I knew they were terrified. "I'm going to be okay," I said hastily. "The plan is that they will just go in and take it all out. Then I won't have cancer anymore." Silence. "It's self-contained, so they just do the hysterectomy and it's gone." They looked horrified. *Good job, Andrea, you didn't cry. Was this the way to say it all? Was I too casual?* How does one know how to share this news with the most cherished of people? "Let's stay here for a bit and talk through all of this so I know that you both understand all of the details and that you're okay."

I looked at them and smiled. I had had two months to digest this news;

this made sharing the facts a little less emotional for me. In hindsight, even though I was careful about how I told them, perhaps I could have been even gentler. I was hoping to come off as not very worried about any of it, hoping that would influence their own reactions.

Maddie looked at me. "Are you scared?"

Yes. Yes, I am. Completely and utterly terrified, actually. The thought of a robotic machine opening me up, cutting up my insides, and then vacuuming them out played through my head non-stop. I kept picturing a hand blender breaking up roasted vegetable soup. I swallowed hard, smiled, and said, "Well, I'm not looking forward to it, but it's done with robotics and is very straightforward, and I have an excellent oncologist doing it. It'll all be fine. So, please, try to understand that this is all nooo biggie. It is only stage one cancer, and they told me that the cells all look fine, so it's not going to be anything major. We're very lucky that we caught it early." I could hear myself blurting it all out a little too quickly. *Had I convinced them I was going to be okay? Had I convinced myself?*

As I was talking, Annie sat there quietly taking it all in, and Maddie studied my face. Both of these young women were highly intuitive and also highly suspicious of me whenever I tried to smooth anything over. They continuously caught on to birthday surprises or a secretly planned trip or anything else I needed to keep hidden.

Almost faltering, I finally finished. Immediately, both of them said, "So what can we do to help? How can we get you through this?"

I was astounded at how mature they both were. *They just received devastating news and yet are thinking past their own emotions and more about mine and how to help me.* I started getting shaky and teary-eyed. I felt so grateful to have these two superstars in my life. The enormous relief of releasing this terrible secret, the challenge and guilt of keeping major news from them for two long months, and the buildup of nerves and worrying about their reactions was all tremendously overpowering and greatly challenged my emotional strength.

I couldn't hold back any longer. I started to cry then, and they immediately stood up and came to me. They became teary too, and I saw them fight a mix of emotions; they didn't want to upset me, yet their own terror was settling deep within. We cried together, holding each other tight, and yet I still felt they were being so very grown up and strong for me. Duey didn't understand what was happening but clearly sensed the tension and saw the emotions. He started barking loudly at us. I wiped my face and blew my nose and said, "I know this is major news, but I think Duey needs to poop. Are we good? I promise you I am not going to die; it'll all be okay." They both nodded, not really able to say much more.

We all knew that Duey didn't need to poop. He is an intuitive dog and a master at reading our emotions. He didn't like that we were crying and he wanted to protect us, to reassure us, and he was upset that we were upset. Nevertheless, we took Duey down to the beach and spent an hour on the shore, jumping out of the way of the icy-cold January waves, collecting shells, and just processing the news. We were all very quiet. I was beyond relieved that I had finally told them and the adrenalin release left me exhausted. After a while we came back inside and I could tell they were both deep in thought, not feeling very good about my news. Soon the time came for them to leave; Maddie had to get to work and Annie had to get home to check on her senior cat. I could tell they didn't want to go. I also didn't want them to leave, but inevitably, with adult kids, that's the way it goes. We hugged for quite a long time, and I reassured them once again that I would be okay. Hesitantly, they left.

I closed the door quietly behind them. Emotionally exhausted and completely broken-hearted, I walked quickly into the bathroom, buried my face in a towel, and cried hard, inconsolable tears.

10
AND BROADER STILL

I eventually came to a place of complete emptiness. Drained both physically and emotionally, I felt nothing and had no more tears to cry. I was glad my daughters finally knew my true situation but I was greatly worried about them. Ultimately, as a mom, my job is to always protect my children. Even while getting through all of this—a life-changing, potentially debilitating disease—my greatest concern was for their well-being.

I thought about who I needed to tell in person. Silently I logged in my head: *two down, a million more to go*. Finally sharing the news with the girls (although stressful and worrisome) was also somewhat relieving, as we had been sitting on this secret for far too long. I had to call my sister, Lara, in California. I texted her and asked if now was a good time to FaceTime her as I had some news.

When I Face Timed her, she was in her car, pulled over, and I simply said, "Okay, are you ready for this?" then took a deep breath. "It's going to blow your mind."

She was all smiles with excitement. "What is it?"

There simply is no easy way of telling people you have cancer. No matter how you set it up, sugar-coated or not, the reaction and shock are still the same. I dropped the hammer. "I have cancer."

I watched her face. It literally fell. Instant shock. All colour drained.

"What?" Her face displaying a myriad of emotions—confusion, disbelief, fear. She started to cry. "Andrea? What? No. No you don't! No!"

I rushed to make things better. "It's only stage one, and it's all coming out in a surgery. It's going to be fine!" I smiled as I stammered. Gosh. I felt so badly telling her.

After a few minutes she pulled herself together and then amazingly, went into big sister mode, asking a million questions, asking me if I needed her to come help, if I had a decent doctor, etc.

I said, "No, the biggest thing I need, is your advice. How on *earth* do we tell Mom?"

As I'd mentioned, Mom was a tough old bird when it came to pain. But emotions? They were a different story altogether. She'd had a lifetime of loss, and I was worried about how emotionally fragile she'd become over the last several years.

Tragically, Mom's first experience of becoming an aunt, such a joyous family time, ended in complete, unexpected tragedy—her sister's baby died when it was only a few days old. Not long after that, Mom's father died of a heart attack; Mom was only in her late twenties.

Several years later, within months of each other, Mom's mother died unexpectedly after a bad flu, and then Mom's second husband died from a heart attack just before their first anniversary. Mom was barely coming up for air when her nephew and later her niece died from substance abuse complications. Heartbreakingly, her golden retriever, a true comfort dog, companion, and best friend of thirteen years, passed away next. All of these events hit her just so hard, with not much time to heal between each unexpected loss. And then only a few years after she lost her dog, her nephew by marriage died of stomach cancer, leaving three young children behind. Less than two years after that, in April 2020, her niece was murdered in the Nova Scotia mass shooting, also leaving behind two young children.

You can well imagine that severe emotional trauma ensued, leaving all of us completely and utterly devastated. Any one of these things was heart-wrenching, but put them all together in a span of only a few years, it's too much for anyone. We witnessed our dear mother trying her hardest to cope, but as each loss came harder and closer together, each more shocking than the last, she became wholly unable to manage. We all needed time, yet time just kept delivering more blows instead of the opportunity to heal.

I felt it was all too fresh to pile on another piece of shattering news only two years after the last tragedy. Nothing could be harder on a mother than to contemplate outliving her child. I told Lara that we really needed to downplay my cancer. I was so afraid of upsetting everyone, I forgot about my own emotions.

In raising our very reactive and emotional mastiff, we learned a term called "stacking." If a dog faces a stress, such as another dog racing over and aggressively barking at him, he reacts, processes, and carries on. If that moment occurs only to be paired with another occurrence (such as a loud city bus zooming noisily by and upsetting him) he would need longer to decompress. If then, a souped-up car revving its noisy engine suddenly sped by, again startling him, followed by an electric scooter whizzing past, and then an unexpected jogger running toward him from around a corner, the dog would now be a primed, nervous bundle of reactivity, ready to jump up and bite the next thing that scares or surprises him. This buildup of events, this "stacking," can wreak havoc on both emotions and nerves in reactive dogs. The same goes for people. Stacking is not good for any creature, human or animal. Our whole family witnessed this as a result of my poor mother's long, unbearable chain of terrible, unexpected, tragic deaths of her loved ones.

I knew I could not put my cancer news off any longer. I drove into town to meet with her. I was truly stressed about disclosing my news; I was afraid this might be the nail in her coffin. To my utmost surprise, Mom took the news rather well. "I knew it," she said. "I just knew it. I have wondered for a very long time." She then nailed me in typical Mom fashion, saying, "You little fibber! You lied to me for months. I had asked you many times if it was cancer, and you told me it wasn't." She sat there, hurt and upset. I had to carefully explain why I was not ready or able to share, not wanting to wreck all of the events in November and December, and most importantly, wanting to tell the girls first.

And so, after I broke the news to Mom, I nervously had to tell my dad, who also had felt his share of loss in the past few years. His second beloved had succumbed to bowel cancer, and he too had to process the huge loss of his dear niece and nephew. I saw that it had greatly affected him, as did the worry for his beloved sister, the mother of his niece and nephew. I was afraid and worried that he too would not be able to cope, and yet, remarkably, he took the news equally well.

After we finished telling the immediate family members, some of our closest friends, and some of my clients, it all felt like it was too much. The anxiety I experienced over and over again as I prepared for peoples' reactions, paired with the very painful aftermath of delivering the blow, was just not something I could continue. Even though it was now ten weeks after I'd received the verdict, I still felt completely overwhelmed and emotionally exhausted by both the diagnosis and the thoughts of the upcoming surgery. (Ten weeks was certainly a long wait living with the knowledge that there was cancer inside me; every day I had to turn off my mind and try not to wonder if the cancer was spreading.)

Ultimately, I decided that for the remaining several people with whom I wanted to share my news, I would choose a very open, honest, and gentle communication through social media. This way, I would be able to summarize and communicate efficiently and effectively and not have to spend hours a week talking about my worrisome health and the details of what was going on. So, mid-January, I shared my diagnosis with the world.

11

THE POWER OF WORDS

Social Media Post #1

January 20

Hello friends ♡

It is time for me to share some tough news. It's about my health. I have been holding this quietly in my heart since November of last year.

After a full year of ups and downs with horrendous symptoms, I finally had a biopsy and learned that I have cancer. (A club I never wanted to join but am now in).

The cancer is an adenocarcinoma, and mine is located in my uterine lining, which can basically be referred to as endometrial cancer. Thankfully it is "only" stage 1, but even knowing that, the weeks of waiting for results and being told that I have cancer, and then more tests to determine the stage and grade, has made life terrifying. ☹

I didn't want anyone to know coming into Christmas time. What a miserable thing to share with family and friends! So, I am sharing this news now, because every single one of you means something to me. ♡ Either you are a new friend whom I love dearly or you are an old friend who I grew up with and also love dearly and share so many happy memories. All of you here bring me great joy, and I love all of you for the positivity and friendship that you offer!

Anyhow, I tell you this news now, because coming up soon, I will go into surgery. I will likely be under for two hours, and I will have a full hysterectomy. For those of you who are not sure what that means, it is the removal of all good stuff. Cervix, ovaries, fallopian tubes, and uterus. It is a big deal to recover from, and I will then be home quietly healing for the next six to eight weeks. (Permission to Netflix binge aaaall daaaaay loooong) ☺ To those of you who feel as though I have fallen off the face of the earth, you now know why!

Looking back, it is funny to see how we appear on Facebook. I know I posted a party picture very recently on New Year's Eve. I literally was in my pyjama bottoms and feeling poorly. However, I said to my husband, let's have some champagne and let's put on some party favours and make a memory because even if we are sad or feeling poorly, it is important to be able to look back at these memories in future times. We will only then see the joy we had for that brief moment.

Hubby has been a rock through this as he and I kept this secret to ourselves for quite a while. My girls, whom I later told, have handled this news with much love, support, and grace. ♡ My sister immediately sent gifts and calls me each day and mom and dad have been champs through all of this; no-one wants to learn their "child" has cancer. My in-laws guide me gently, as they are with much experience in this disease and have provided much encouragement and knowledge. My besties and all of my guitar friends have been incredibly nurturing, and my circle has been hugely supportive toward me. I feel well loved and well looked after. ♡

Anyhow, that is all for now. I do hope in the next week or so that any of you who believes in prayer or meditation / positive vibes can send a few my way as I prepare for this next part of the process. The surgery makes me nervous, but I'm also excited to hopefully put this all behind me soon. They will do a biopsy while I'm under and hopefully two weeks after that (likely around Valentine's Day) ♡ I will know whether or not they got all of it out! So, if you also would like to say a good prayer for it to have contained itself, I would really appreciate it.

That is all. Be well and be kind to one another. I love you all so much ♡

To my complete and utter surprise, I had 399 comments that afternoon and several hundred phone calls, emails, and texts in the days following. I spoke with people I hadn't heard from in years, and I was truly overjoyed and amazed by the sheer volume of people who had reached out. I had no idea I would have such huge support and love coming back to me.

From a lifetime of confusion and struggles (and the aftermath of those struggles all from unmanaged ADHD), admittedly, I had no sense of self-worth. The huge outpouring of love and support through phone calls and visits was immensely helpful and equalled only by the purely magnificent power of the written words; they carried me through the next several weeks.

And so, this troubling, challenging time was the beginning not only of a physical journey to healing, but also of an emotional one. I sincerely believe I am deeply and unquestionably changed by each and every person who connected with me, and for that I am eternally grateful.

12

ALL BOOKED AND GOOD TO GO

A few days after making my social media post, I received a phone call from the booking office. "Andrea?" a loud voice asked, it was not a familiar one.

"Yes?" I replied, already walking over to grab a paper and pen.

"This is the booking office. I have your surgery date. Are you ready to take down the information?"

"Yes." My heart started to pound. *This is happening.*

"The surgery will be February first."

Finally. "Okay. This is for my hysterectomy, right?" I asked, feeling foolish. *You never can be too careful these days.*

"Yes, that's right. Did you have another surgery coming up besides this one?"

"Uh, no," I replied. One time I thought I had a podiatrist appointment for my plantar fasciitis, and I showed up to the address with my toes all freshly manicured only to walk into my long-awaited proctology appointment. I was pretty surprised when I was told to drop my drawers.

"Are you writing this down?" the voice asked.

My brain started to feel like when you eat ice cream too fast.

"Make sure you pack a comfort bag. You will want that after the surgery.

Toothbrush, slippers, and gum. Lots of gum. You will need to chew gum to stimulate your bowels."

"Okay, got it. And where do I go?" I asked, feeling like the other information was self-explanatory and that she needed to start with the more important wheres and whens.

"February first, Dickson Building. You need to be there for 6:30 a.m."

Oh gosh that will mean an early start coming in from Peggy's Cove.

"Oh, you should also know that you are not going to have Dr. blah-bitty-blah, you will have Dr. Stephanie Scott instead."

A big pause as I panicked and could not speak. "Wait! Wh-why the change?" I had already met with the other surgeon and had talked through my concerns and questions. I didn't feel comfortable at the thought of a complete stranger operating on me.

"She's away on vacation," the voice said.

Well crap. That is not good. "I guess I can understand that," I replied, trying to sound calm.

We spoke in greater detail on the early time, arrival, where to go, what else to bring, etc. I carefully jotted it all down and reviewed it all after we'd hung up.

"Who was that?" Mike asked.

I swallowed hard, feeling a little shaky. "That was the booking office. My surgery is on February first." *Two weeks from today.* I hurriedly googled the name of the newly assigned surgeon. She had good reviews and from the few pics I found online it appeared as though she was a fairly "normal" person. That was a big relief.

I had two weeks to get ready. Two weeks to get the house in order; we'd only been living there for just under three months. It was mid-January and we were still unpacking items from storage and still had a few Christmas things up. I certainly would not be up and moving or lifting for a good eight weeks after the surgery, and I dove in to the task of more in-depth house organizing as best I could. It helped keep my mind off things.

Once I felt that the house was more manageable, I carefully researched and packed every comfort item I could think of to get me through the surgery and what I might like to have in recovery later that day through my hospital stay. I packed water bottles, mints, gum, nourishing snacks, my favourite slippers, a cozy bathrobe, a blanket, my teddy bear, a cellphone charger, toothbrush, mouthwash, a hairbrush, lip balm, a Sudoku puzzle book, and a few other miscellaneous items. I put my clean underwear right at the top of the bag.

In hindsight, I should've packed a gun.

13

THE DAYS LEADING UP
TO THE BIG EVICTION

With the hysterectomy coming up, there were tests, tests, and more tests. One day a call came in and I was informed that I needed to get a CT scan done in preparation for the surgery. I'd had one back in November just after the initial diagnosis, but another one was needed for some reason. Now, I'd always prided myself on being mentally strong; able to power through adversity. It is, however, interesting to come to understand the power of the body when *it* makes the decision on how to handle things, instead of the conscious mind.

In the weeks prior to this particular morning's appointment, I had had several blood tests. I was starting to notice that my body didn't like needles very much. I was definitely not powering through when I was poked more than a few times. All my life, I'd scoffed at people who said they'd faint at the sight of blood, needles, or when getting blood work. I truly thought they were wimps, mainly because they would get so worked up about the whole thing beforehand. You can imagine my complete surprise when, on this day while getting the IV set up for the scan, my body completely turned against me. My brain was confident, but my body decided to conduct things quite differently, and it fully exposed my vulnerabilities.

At this point, I still walked in to my appointments and treatments with confidence. Yes, I felt some jitters, but that was normal. I had not experienced much trouble with any diagnostics or treatments yet, so today I naively expected things to still go smoothly. Each time there was an interaction, I made a point of being polite, patient, trusting, and accepting with the various staff and all of the required procedures.

When I arrived at the hospital for the scan, a nurse brought me to a room to set up the necessary IV. I learned that not all CT scans required an IV and contrast dye, but this one did. Information was needed to thoroughly examine, measure, and prepare for the upcoming operation with the "full" hysterectomy. Consequently, careful measurements and accurate information must be acquired in order to prepare for each individual's procedure.

A young nurse greeted me in the dimly lit room in which I awaited setup. She seemed a little awkward and quite unsure of herself, and I suspect this was the beginning of my subsequent reaction. If someone lacks confidence, that suggests to me that they are not very good at what they do and it's quite worrisome thinking one is not in good hands for these types of things. Being keenly aware of people's body language and what it indicates can make me anxious and uneasy. At times, it's a bit of a curse.

The nurse got out the needed items for the IV, carefully placed my arm in her lap, and began looking for a vein. She still seemed a little uncertain as she attempted to insert the needle. Immediately I felt a sharp, searing pain. I jumped. She jumped. She looked up at me in surprise and then started to blush. "Whoops." she said. "Sorry about that. They usually seem to just go right in." I smiled calmly and reassured her that I was okay. I felt badly for her awkwardness and didn't want to be the one to scar her for life with my big reaction, potentially causing anxiety in her when she had to set up future IVs. I tried to remain calm. She tried again.

"Ow!" I yelled. This time the skin on my arm turned bright red as blood quickly escaped.

She looked horrified and turned an odd shade of green. "I'll b-be right back," she stammered. She exited quickly. She was not *right back* at all. A full ten minutes passed as I sat in the chair waiting and wondering what was going on.

A second, older nurse came in. "You Andrea?" she quickly asked.

"Yup." I smiled, although now slightly less enthusiastic. "That's me."

"Okay, well I'm here to try to get the IV in you. I guess you don't got good veins?" she said, with a sort of half smile and an odd look. And then she shrugged like she was up for a challenge.

I found her body language confusing. "Uh, I guess that depends on who's trying to access them?" I joked.

She didn't really react to that and methodically began looking for a good vein. She spent several minutes looking. For some reason, before even her first attempt, my mind started telling me she was going to hurt me. In those few seconds before she began, I fought and reasoned with myself and felt like I had won.

Interrupting my thoughts, she said "Okay, I think I found one. I'm goin' in." She bit her lower lip and her shoulders rose up to her ears.

Now, it's one thing to have a nurse who is not good at inserting needles and a little nervous, but it is a complete other thing to have a nurse who is not very good at needles who is reckless and completely oblivious to the pain being caused. She poked. It pinched. Again I felt a searing hot pain in my arm.

"Darn it!" she exhaled. "I thought I had it." She wiggled the needle around inside my arm. I could feel it moving. "This little frigger isn't gettin' away today!" she announced. I honestly felt like she thought she was casting a line trying to hook a fish. "You got real roly veins, don't cha?" I began to feel nauseated. "Shoot!" She sounded annoyed now. "I only get two tries. Hang on there." She was determined to get it, as she didn't want to leave the room having failed. I began to feel faint.

"How about we take a break?" I suggested, smiling at her. She looked up, surprised, like she had no idea she was hurting me.

"Oh. Okay." She pulled the needle out as I turned my head away. "What, you don't like 'em?" she asked.

"It just helps me if I don't actually look," I said quietly. I could feel my heart rate speeding up, and my fingers started to feel numb.

I tried to slow my breathing and think happy thoughts. My mind went to a sunny beach in Cuba, and I imagined a healthy, tanned version of me doing the limbo while handsome men cheered me on. I could hear the tune of the limbo playing in my head. *Lul-lul la- la la- la la . . .* I stayed in that scene for the next few minutes, fighting hard not to feel upset. *Lul-lul la- la la- la la . . .*

"Oh for heaven's sake," I heard. I opened my eyes. She had dropped the needle on the floor. She stood up, left the room, quickly returned with a new set of items, and rushed the next attempt.

Again, searing pain. "Ow!" I yelled.

She looked up. She seemed almost angry, as if I was deliberately giving her a hard time.

"Sorry," I apologized, and again, smiled. She looked like she was about to attempt a *third* time and I intervened. "Two's the rule, right?" I stated, looking directly at her. She looked like she was going to overrule the rule for a second, and I jumped in again and said, "So, who's next?"

She sighed, visibly disappointed and frustrated. Slowly she stood, stared at me a moment, and then saying nothing, abruptly left.

Maybe it was the release of tension paired with the huge volume of adrenalin, but just as she exited, my body decided it had had enough. I started seeing long, black, cylindrical tunnels, and I felt like I was spinning out of control. *Is my blood pressure rapidly dropping?*

Being alone in a strange environment when you're about to faint is no fun at all. I was unfamiliar at that point with the physical symptoms of fainting but knew I was feeling dangerously unwell and totally vulnerable. Silently, I coached myself. *You got this, Andrea. Breathe slowly. You're okay.*

I fought the feelings for several seconds and then started panting heavily as I broke into a sweat. "Hello?" I called. I waited. Nothing. I started to really struggle and began to feel slumpy. "Hello!" I called again. Still nothing. I could hear people talking just beyond the door, so I knew they were nearby. "Hello! I need help!" I yelled it very loudly this time in my big, band teacher voice that I tended to use when conducting junior high kids honking away on various unpracticed instruments. The voices stopped.

"Did that come from in there?" I heard someone say.

"Yes!" I yelled, hoping they had nodded at my door and that I hadn't just redirected them elsewhere.

Just as I started to faint, three nurses rushed in to see what was happening. I felt my body collapse in the chair and then hands were on me, putting my chair back and my feet up. A cold washcloth was placed on my forehead. "You're okay, we're here." a voice said reassuringly. I breathed in, slowly, deeply. I was so annoyed by all of this. "We will get that IV in, in just a few minutes. You just relax, okay?" *Relax? Oh the irony of that statement.* Even though I felt like crap, my brain still had some retorts that I wisely chose to keep to myself.

After a few minutes in my still fragile state, a fourth nurse entered the room and successfully got the IV in. Huge relief. They wheeled me into the CT room and I weakly transferred myself from the chair to the table to go into the giant grey machine. The large grey circle made me think of a doughnut, or a Lifesaver candy. *They really should paint something fun on that circle,* I thought. *A pink doughnut with sprinkles or something yummy. Wouldn't that make it so much better? "How was your day today?" someone might ask, and you could say, "Oh it was awesome! I was inside a large, frosted pink, sprinkly doughnut for my CT scan!"* I mean, really, they could do that, to make these processes a little better; it's not rocket science.

Because I have claustrophobia, I knew to close my eyes before the machine moved me in to the tight little tunnel. Music played softly and I felt people adjusting me. "Hands over your head please," a voice commanded. I quickly did as I was told. I liked the music at least, and I mentioned that. Maybe it's the teacher in me, but positive feedback is always important. The bed started moving and in I went. "Big breath in . . . hold . . . and release." The commanding voice said this phrase several more times and then finally I heard, "Okay, Andrea, we are going to put the dye in now. Let us know right away if you feel uncomfortable, okay?"

Great, I thought, *I hope I'm not allergic to this.* "Okay!" I sang out. I tried to hide my anxiety, like this was no big deal. I have multiple allergies, so inside that tunnel I was secretly, silently praying.

Warm liquid zapped into my arm, and about ten seconds later I felt like

I had peed. *Oh my gosh! Why the heck did I just pee? How am I going to walk out of here with pee all over my legs and a soaking wet johnnie shirt?*

That very awkward incident brought me back to another childhood memory . . . this time, I was in grade four. My mom had signed me up to join the Girl Guides of Canada; Bedford, Nova Scotia troupe. I was surprised she had done that as I'd failed miserably in Brownies; a lower aged group before Girl Guides. For some reason, I was the Brownie with no badges and always had a messy uniform. I was certain that Girl Guides was not really my thing but Mom felt it would be good for me.

The meetings were held at a church with which I was unfamiliar. Dad diligently drove me over on that first night; I was dressed in my cobalt blue uniform and polyester scarf. As usual, we had been late leaving the house and I had had no time to use the bathroom. When we got to the church, I told Dad that I had to pee. Dad glanced at me and casually suggested, "Just ask them when you get in there, where the bathroom is." To an adult, that sounded straight forward enough, but to a kid who was overwhelmed and not yet socially confident, it was not a great suggestion.

I bravely walked into the church hall, looked around and realized I didn't know a soul. Girls ran around hugging each other and screaming in excitement as adult leaders organized flags for the various older Guides to hold. It was sheer chaos as apparently everyone in the pack knew each other and this was the first night back after the summer hiatus. I didn't feel comfortable asking a stranger where the bathroom was and I mistakenly decided to hold it.

Out of the blue, someone yelled a command and the girls fell neatly into several rows of four and began marching on the spot. I scrambled to join in and tried to get my feet to march on the same count as theirs. Like windshield wipers that don't match the speed of others, I couldn't figure out how to fall in line. I didn't know that if I'd just repeated the same leg coming up that the cycle would correct itself, but it didn't matter, I had to pee so badly now my legs were going up and down much faster than theirs anyhow. I was so desperate to use the bathroom, I began squirming.

Much like getting a heavy army tank going, the troup started moving slowly in a circle, each Girl Guide carefully taking small steps forward so as not to step on the heels of those in front of them. Gradually they picked up speed. I heard the robust singing of "Oh Canada" and I joined in; trying my hardest to march, move and sing our National Anthem. My bladder felt ready to burst and I desperately searched the walls for a bathroom sign. *None anywhere!* Touted flags gently flowed as we marched in a large circle and I became more and more desperate. My legs were now doing double time, my feet hopping along in a fast squirmy dance.

And then to my complete horror, it happened. My bladder burst. Just like that, warm pee flowed down my legs, filled my shoes and spilled over onto the floor. *Oh no.* I thought. *What am I going to do?* The Guides continued marching, oblivious to my situation. A second thought occurred. *Perfect!* I reasoned, *I'll march along and I won't be anywhere near the pee puddle!* I smiled to myself, half relieved, but in my panic, I hadn't completely thought this through. As we were all marching, it meant that ultimately it would not be a puddle around me, but rather a trail. Everyone in the room was going to march right through the pee as it continued to flow down my now thoroughly saturated tights while I was still in motion.

Girl Guides happily sang the Anthem, as every single shoe behind me marched and tracked urine along the inner part of the circle. At this point, no one had yet noticed; they were all with eyes on the flags and singing loudly and proudly. Finally, I finished peeing. My legs were warm and my shoes were soaked. *I had gotten away with it!* I relaxed and smiled to myself. *Now, if I could only remain comfortable enough to get through the next hour and a half, I could go home and no one would ever know.* I loved the pretty, colorful, flowy flags and the singing of Oh Canada. *I might just come to like girl guides after all!* I thought.

And, just as I believed I would make it out alive, very abruptly, I heard mass confusion as people saw the mess on the floor. "Is there a leak?" someone asked. "Where did all of this water come from?" someone else now inquired, a little louder. "What is this?" someone said, as they looked at the faintly yellowish hue. Worriedly I looked around. It really *was* tracked all over the entire hall. People started looking at each other, questioning what had happened. As it quickly dawned on me in realization that I could be found out, my face betrayed me. I started blushing. I lowered my head so no one would see my now beet red face and I prayed silently. *"Don't let them know it's me. Don't let them know it's me!"* I repeated this mantra over and over.

In a flash, the jig was up. "It's pee!" I heard someone yell. "EWW!" several more voices joined in . . . I heard almost every single person react loudly in disgust. "I walked in pee!" others cried mournfully. Again, sheer chaos. The leaders, in panic, looked hastily around the room and then one leader caught my eye. She knew instantly that I had done this. She walked toward me as the Girl Guides tracked her. Their eyes ultimately landed on the trembling, teary, red-faced new girl. "She's the one! She peed!" they all started to yell.

To my absolute horror, they pointed directly at me. I didn't know where the doors were in this new place and could not escape. I stood there, trembling quite violently, crying full out sobs. The leader finally made it over to me and directed me out to a black pay phone on the wall. My legs were stiff and robotic-like from full adrenaline.

"Would you like to call someone to come get you?" she whispered. "Yes." I replied, still shaking. She reached into her tiny brown leather purse that was attached to her skinny brown leather belt. She passed me a dime, and that was that. She left the room and I put my trembling fingers into the little holes of the rotary dial, cursing the numbers in my phone number as I waited for each revolution.

Dad answered. "Helloo?" he crooned. "Come get me" I said. In those days you never knew who was calling; there were no screens or identifiers. It took him a few seconds to clue in that it was me. "What?" he asked. He had just arrived home from dropping me off. "Why?" In complete and utter exasperation, I replied, "BECAUSE I JUST PEED EVERYWHERE AND I AM NEVER GOING BACK TO GUIDES AGAIN!" I hung up the phone. I didn't wait for an answer or a debate or any further questions.

After what seemed like forever, Dad's car finally pulled in. I ran out as fast as my wet legs could take me and to my embarrassment saw that he had carefully lined the fabric seats of the car with black garbage bags. I looked at him, eyes questioning. "Well," he stammered sheepishly, "I didn't want you to stink up the car."

Bright lights came on and I heard people's voices. "All done Andrea. Can we help you up?" I was back in the CT scan room.

"Uh," I blurted, "I think I might've peed." I was completely horrified.

"Oh, not likely. That is a common sensation from the dye. You're alright!"

What? Really? Gosh I hope they're right. I didn't really believe them until I actually got up and, to my utter relief, they were correct. I was perfectly dry.

14

THE BIG DAY

The two weeks sped by and the morning of the surgery came early. I was going on very little sleep, as I was nervous about the new surgeon and scared of the invasive procedures. To picture myself with legs spread-eagled in the air on an operating table, unconscious, and with a tube down my throat while strangers cut into me and pulled things out was absolutely terrifying. *What if I'm not completely knocked out? What if I wake up during the surgery and no one realizes? What if there are complications and I bleed out?* I was paralyzed with fear as my mind raced out of control.

We made the long drive in silence and I had way too much time to think about all of the what-ifs. Finally, we pulled up to the hospital. "Well, here we are. Do you want me to park first or drop you off first?" Mike smiled at me and placed his hand on mine.

"I don't know," I quietly said. I couldn't even make that decision. Cars were lining up behind us as I looked at him, my mind frozen.

"Okay, in you go. I'll park and come find you. You're gonna be okay."

I almost cried but tried my hardest to look brave. "Okay" is all I could muster, my lips quivering, and I got out of the car.

I walked to the elevator with my bag and followed the directions on my paper. I arrived at check-in and the nurse handed me a blue-striped johnnie shirt, a mint-green robe, a hair cover that resembled a bag, and puffy paper slippers. The room was filled with several other overtired, nervous people, all of us likely feeling vulnerable and worried. "Go get changed and leave your bag on the trolley over there," the nurse said gruffly.

"What happens to it then?" I politely asked.

"It'll be brought to you after surgery," she said, a little less gruffly.

I followed the orders but debated what to do with my cellphone. I decided to put it safely hidden in my bag, and apprehensively I walked to the waiting room again. Mike showed up and I was aware of my body slumping in relief when I saw him. He was about to sit down when they called my name. I looked at him in panic. I looked at the lady with the clipboard. "Can he come with me?" I asked quickly, my stomach tying itself in knots.

"Nope," she replied, just as gruffly as the other nurse. Clearly these people were used to dealing with whiners and beggars, and they cut them off at the knees. "From this point onward it's just you."

I was hugely disappointed. I thought Mike would be waiting with me until the surgery time at 8:00. It was only 6:45. My spirits sank. I turned to him and smiled, trying to be brave one last time. He gave me a big hug and said, "I love you. You're gonna be fine."

I turned and followed the clipboard lady and was aware of five or six others who had joined the group, nervously following along. *Ha. We are all being corralled like sheep to the slaughter.*

I was given a stretcher to lie on in a hallway and was covered in warm flannel sheets. I curled up and closed my eyes. Amazingly, I actually dozed off.

"Andrea?" A gentle voice spoke my name and my eyes flew open. I saw a warm hearted face wearing a surgical mask, looking down at me. "I am Dr. Scott."

"You are?" I said in wonder, awe, and relief. She was lovely.

"Yes." She smiled. "I am. How are you doing?" she asked sweetly.

I almost cried then; she was so kind and caring. "To be truthful, I'm really scared." I tried to keep my lower lip from trembling.

She reached down and patted my arm. "That's understandable. We are going to take good care of you. I promise." I got teary-eyed. "Do you have any questions before we go in?" She smiled at me again. I told her my concerns about the anesthetic and she reassured me the anesthesiologist in the O.R. was really good and that I would be just fine.

We spoke for another few minutes and then she left me so she could get prepped for the surgery. I settled into the idea that this might actually turn out okay. I closed my eyes and dozed off again and then woke to a young man calling my name and telling me I had to get up and off the stretcher and walk into the operating room. He offered me his arm like he was my prom date. I almost joked about it but was not feeling up to being funny.

In we went. The room was brightly lit and there were about five people dressed in light-blue scrubs and masks. Music played in the background and they showed me what to do to get up on the table. They belted me in and the anesthesiologist looked down at me with big brown eyes and a gigantic smile. "How's Miss Andrea doin' today!" He spoke with a lilting Jamaican accent.

"I'm okay. Just make sure you really knock me out well, okay?" I pleaded.

He laughed. "All 'da red-heads want 'da big drugs, don't they?" He placed a mask over my face and instructed me to breathe in slowly. He counted down and in five seconds I was out cold.

15

NURSE LOVELY, NURSE SMILEY, AND THE EVIL WITCH FROM HELL

I woke up from surgery high as a kite. I was thrilled that I was only just now conscious and that I hadn't woken up in the middle of surgery as I had feared. I looked around. There were six or seven other patients all recovering in the large hospital room. I noted that I felt hungry and also wondered how my procedure had gone in the O.R. I also wondered what time of day it was.

A cheerful young nurse came over to my bed. "Well hello, Andrea." She smiled. "How are you doing?" I tried to speak but my mouth was dry and my voice wouldn't come out. "Oh, I bet you need some water. Or in fact, would you like a Popsicle?" I nodded. She brought over a bright green Popsicle. I weakly brought it to my lips. *Lime. So good!* I hadn't eaten since eight o'clock the night before.

"Thank you," I croaked. "What time is it?" My voice was weak and odd-sounding.

"You're probably feeling the effects of the tube," she said kindly. "It's three p.m."

I stared at her, as I couldn't figure out what day it was. "Is it still today?"

I asked. I meant was this only a few hours post-op. I couldn't get my brain to figure out how to ask that. She laughed. She knew what I meant.

"Yes. It is still today."

I sucked on that Popsicle like it was highly sought-after rain-water collected in a desert leaf. I was indeed thirsty, and famished.

She watched me closely. "I see that you're hungry. Would you like another Popsicle?"

I nodded.

"And how is the pain? I have pain meds for you."

I weakly replied that I was sore, and she immediately left and came back in a flash with pain meds and more Popsicles. She stayed by my side while I devoured the next one. She was really kind. As it was not very busy in the recovery room, she stayed with me for quite a while. We talked about many things and ultimately got around to our pets. I told her all about Duey. My pain started to become intense and I didn't feel like whatever she gave me was working. She looked concerned for me.

"Those meds should have kicked in by now." She frowned. Next she asked me what narcotics I had had in the past, and she explained that sometimes it takes a bit of experimenting to get the right combo and the right amounts to work most effectively. She came back with something else and I took it. She added something to my IV. Immediately I felt relief. "How's that?" she asked, with her hand gently on my arm.

"Better." I smiled. I was grateful for her thoughtfulness. She was a wonderful and caring nurse.

"So, your catheter was removed, but we need to get you to pee before we send you to your hospital room. Do you think you can pee?"

I looked at her, sort of confused. *How would I ever manage to get to a toilet?*

She must've realized what I was thinking and explained, "Don't worry, I'm going to bring you a hat."

I didn't know what a hat was for and reasoned it likely to be a medical term for something. "Okay." I croaked again. My throat was really sore.

I swear there must have been two of her because quick as a flash she was gone and back. She held a white plastic container with wings on the side. It resembled a top hat. I looked at it and then at her. *How on earth would I pee in that?*

"Okay," she said, "I'm going to slide this under you. Can you raise your bum?"

Good grief. I had to pee in front of her? What if I missed the pot? What if I got it in the bed? Or down my back? Or—oh my gosh—on her HAND? I was, and I am not exaggerating, *totally* horrified to consider this task as vivid Girl Guide memories came flooding back to me in my medically-induced-high state.

She laughed again. "It's okay. This is what we do up here with everyone, every day, all the time." God love her, she truly was a saint.

"Okay. I'm really sorry to do this to you," I said, embarrassed.

"On the count of three, lift your bum." This was almost impossible to do. I was weak and sore and quite high on drugs. She counted and on three I grunted and heaved and ultimately managed to lift up my bum. With lightening-speed, she thrust the hat under my pelvis. Of course, completely pee shy, nothing happened. I waited. *C'mon, Andrea, pee!* I thought. My legs started to shake as the effort to keep my pelvis raised in this half-bridge with my feet slipping on the sheets was beginning to exhaust me. Still no pee. Finally, a little dribble. *Ouch.* The pain from having a catheter in for several hours during and post-surgery was making things sting. Finally, after a great amount of effort, a long stream came out. My knees were slamming hard together and I could no longer keep myself raised. All of a sudden my butt came crashing down without warning as my feet shot out from underneath me. She deftly grabbed the pee hat and got it out from under me just in time. She cracked up laughing. "Whoa! That was a close one! Well done. We didn't spill a drop."

Totally embarrassed, I smiled at her again, dreamily. "You are the loveliest person I have ever met."

She smiled and said, "Well aren't you the kindest. Thank you."

As I drifted in and out of sleep, I was faintly aware of patients coming and going in their recovery beds. I was the only one that wasn't being wheeled out. I asked Nurse Lovely if I could have my bag. I wanted my Vaseline for my dry lips, my cellphone, and some gum. I recalled they had said to chew gum as much as possible to get your bowels moving; later I would learn the true importance of this. Nurse Lovely explained that my bag had been brought down to my room already and we were just waiting on the doctor to see me and then I would be transferred. I was getting anxious to check text messages and to tell my daughters I was okay. I missed my husband and wanted to hear his voice.

"I can bring you a portable phone if you want to make some calls." She had read my mind. Zip! She speedily returned with an old grey phone. She dialed for me. No answer. I was really disappointed. *Why was Mike not answering?* Just then I looked up, and lo and behold, he was right beside me. I blinked. My hunny-bunny was right there! I couldn't believe it.

"Is this real?" I asked deliriously. "Am I dreaming or are you really here?"

He laughed and gave me a great smile. "It's real. I'm here." He hugged me, a great big bear hug. He looked relieved.

"Oh my gosh." I smiled a druggy smile. "I love you soooo much." I started crying tears of relief and joy. This man is my rock.

Mike chuckled. "I'm not supposed to be in here. I'll come back when you have your room and are settled. Where's your phone?" He wanted to make sure I had what I needed.

"It's in my bag in my room, waiting for me."

"Okay. Call me when you get settled and I'll be right over. Okay, love you, bye." Kiss-kiss.

He left and the nurse said, "We're not really supposed to have visitors up here, but I know how badly you wanted to see him."

All of a sudden my heavenly angel oncologist surgeon, whom I had only just met that morning, came in, all smiles. "Hi, Andrea." She waved as she walked over to me. "You are doing great. The surgery went well. I got everything out and I feel like that's it. You should be through this nightmare once you're all healed up from surgery. We can't say for sure, of course, until the pathology comes back, but I feel pretty optimistic about it all."

That was the best news! I was so, so glad and so very relieved, I started crying. Until you are faced with the risk of a deadly disease lying in the wings, you won't really grasp the immense amount of stress I was under up until that very moment. I had gone three long, full months worrying and trying my hardest to deal with the deep concern I had, waiting for the confirmation in this very moment. Three months is a looong wait. She took my hand in hers. She gave it a squeeze. There was something so very special and kind in her eyes. She was a brilliant, determined, strong woman, and I felt so well cared for. I immediately trusted her and felt a connection to her like we had known one another in a past life. I thanked her profusely for her excellent care and squeezed her hand.

She smiled. "Okay, get some rest. I'll call your husband and let him know how you are doing, and I'll be back to check on you in the morning."

She called Mike on the phone right by my bedside and again I heard her say everything looked great and went well. She was quite happy about it all. I fell asleep again, exhausted and enormously relieved.

At six o'clock on the dot I woke up in a great deal of pain. I was surprised to see that I was still in the recovery room, yet this time with a different staff. I was the only patient still there. Another kind nurse was immediately by my side.

"Right on time." She smiled. "Your pain meds last for three hours, and you are due for some more." She had them ready and I swallowed them quickly. My stomach growled loudly. "You must be hungry," she said. "When did you eat last?"

I thought for a moment. "Eight o'clock."

"Last night?" She was a little surprised. "As in twenty-two hours ago?"

"Yes," I confirmed. "But I had two Popsicles."

She looked at me apologetically. "We have no food here in recovery besides Popsicles, but you will be brought down soon. We have called a few times asking when they will be ready for you, and they said they are waiting on a room. You will not be on the cancer recovery floor, though, as they are already full. You will be on the sixth floor and we will bring you down just as soon as we can."

Too hungry to sleep, I looked around and realized that it was only the two of us now in the room. I really wanted my bag. It had my snacks, my phone, and all the comforts I was missing: hand cream, my teddy bear, a cozy blanket, and slippers. I felt really out of touch and wanted to call my girls and text my mom and sister. I knew Mike was waiting to come back to see me tonight before his long drive back to our home on the ocean. I asked again about the bag and was assured that as soon as I was settled in my room, my bag would be there.

Just then, to my surprise, Mike appeared. I was so relieved. He gave me another huge hug. He had had dinner with his father and wanted to see that I was settled. He too was surprised that I was still in recovery. He explained that he needed to go as Duey had been left alone in his crate for far too many hours, and although I was disappointed, I put on a brave face as I knew Duey needed food and water and to be let outside to do his business. Mike asked me if I was okay. I smiled and said yes, but truly, I was worried about my pain, the stitches and my recovery. The plan was to pick me up the next morning to bring me home.

"Have you talked with Annie and Maddie?" I asked.

"Yes. I told them everything is fine and that you made out just great."

"Okay." I smiled weakly. "I can manage. You go."

He gave me a squeeze and quietly left.

Nurse Smiley pulled up a chair and sat with me. We ended up talking for quite a long time. It was a moment reminiscent of my youth, when in some random bar bathroom, you meet a stranger and immediately bond. Great, life-altering conversations are had but by the next morning you cannot, for the life of you, recollect any of them. Nurse Smiley and I had life all figured out in my narcotic euphoria, but by eight thirty I started having more discomfort and asked for some more pain relief.

"I'm so sorry, sweetie," she said. "You have to try and make it to nine p.m. It's just half an hour; do you think you can hang on?"

I felt a little panicked, as the pain was quite uncomfortable, but I nodded. I could do it. I watched the clock. At 8:55 the old desk phone rang and I overheard my nurse discussing a room number and plan. She hung up and exclaimed happily, "Good news! We will bring you down now."

I asked if I could now have my meds and she explained that the porters were on their way and I would get my meds in my new room. I was getting more and more uncomfortable. At 9:10 the porters finally showed up. They were large, strong men who liked to joke around. They were able to distract me enough that I made it to the sixth floor without moaning, but I was getting desperate now for the pain meds.

They rolled me down the hallway, and the bed banged and rocked as they tried to get it into the room. The motion and jerking of the bed on my tender surgical site left me in deep pain even though they were trying to be careful. Ultimately they got the large bed in there. The room was dark and smelled very stale.

I carefully whispered, "Are there others in this room?" (I had asked for a private.)

"Yes, there are three others."

"Okay," I whispered again. I didn't want to wake anyone.

They left and I was alone in the dark wondering what to do and how to get a nurse.

"Hello?" I whispered. Nothing. "Hello?" I whispered a little louder. Nothing. I found a buzzer by my bed and pressed it.

I heard an angry voice. "What?"

"Uh, can a nurse come see me please?" I feebly asked, trying not to disturb anyone in the room.

"Just a minute," the voice barked on the other end.

I was now really uncomfortable, and a deep pain in my belly had started. In great agony and trying not to cry, I waited for the nurse. I looked at the clock on the wall. Five minutes passed. Ten. I began squirming, unable to lay still from the pain of surgery and sweating from the effort to control the aching. Finally, the nurse arrived. She entered loudly and left the heavy door open. Bright lights from the hallway lit up my area.

"What do you want?" she snapped. I was shocked.

"I need my meds." I groaned.

"What meds?" she snapped again.

"I was supposed to have my pain meds at nine o'clock. I really need them, I'm quite uncomfortable." I tried to sound kind and patient.

"Who told you that?" She frowned and I saw deep lines in her forehead.

"The nurse upstairs in recovery told me that. She said it's every three hours and I've been in pain since eight thirty. She said I had to wait till nine to get them. I know it's well after nine. I'm in a lot of pain." I tried to explain things clearly and gently. I was surprised by her demeanour.

"Well. That's not how it works down here. It's every *four* hours. You have to wait till ten." She turned on her heel and started to leave.

"Wait!" I said. "I still need my bag."

"What bag?" she snapped again.

I explained that I had been told that my bag would be here and that I needed it.

"I don't know what you're talking about," she said. "There's no bag here."

With that, she left. I was speechless. I started to cry. I was in agonizing pain, and I needed help. I was hungry, quite astonished by the behaviour of this nurse, exhausted, and losing my patience. I had been waiting six hours now for my cellphone and just needed to get comfortable.

I started to breathe too fast as the pain became unbearable. I broke out in another wave of sweat, realizing that my hormones were taking a nose-dive with my ovaries now removed. I tried my absolute hardest to count the minutes to get to ten o'clock but could no longer deal with the pain, and so I desperately buzzed the nurse again. I asked her about the meds. She said she was bringing them. Relieved, I lay quietly in the dark. I waited and waited and waited, starting to uncontrollably whimper aloud. I pressed my lips together hard to keep from crying out. I didn't want to wake the others, but it was too much. I started full on crying. Ultimately the same crabby nurse came back in.

"What are you doing?" she asked loudly.

"What?" I looked at her in confusion.

"You are crying. What is wrong?"

"I am in a great deal of pain from the surgery, my chest hurts and I am desperate for my meds."

She looked at me with disgust. "Andrea," she said patronizingly, "you had a hysterectomy. You're not dying. There are people in here with holes in their stomach dying of cancer. You're going home in the morning, you're fine."

My jaw dropped in disbelief. Did she even know my surgery *was* to remove cancer? She handed me my meds in a small paper cup. I looked at her, waiting for the Styrofoam water cup to follow.

"What?" she snapped again. *Is this the only way she knows how to talk?*

"Could I please have some water to swallow the pills?" I feebly requested.

She looked at me, sighing, and replied angrily, "You don't have any water?"

I explained I had packed water bottles in my bag but that I was still waiting for it. She left and came back with half a cup of water, just barely enough for me to get the pills down. The hospital curtain was now blocking the clock. I asked her what time it was.

"Ten thirty," she said, curtly.

I gasped. Now two hours past the time when I first desperately needed the pain meds, over twenty-six hours since I had had solid food, and ample time for my bag to be located but yet it was still missing, I started to feel quite worried about my situation.

I recalled Nurse Smiley explaining that they would have food to give me once I got to my room. My stomach, once again, loudly made itself known. Feeling quite weak, I struggled to get my words out and feared the wrath that my request might elicit. I asked anyway as I was so very desperate. "Can I have something to eat please?"

She slowly turned her head. I swear she had hate in her eyes. "It's ten thirty p.m., Andrea. You can't wait till the morning?" She clearly did not want to do any work.

Baffled, I looked at her and explained as patiently as I could, "I have not eaten in twenty-six hours."

She stared at me for a moment. "Well, I cannot give you anything. This isn't the floor that has food. That's the cancer floor. You are not *on* that floor."

I couldn't believe my ears. I begged. "A piece of toast? Do you have toast?"

"Yes," she answered reluctantly. "I will make you toast."

"And can you please locate my bag?" I asked.

"Andrea, I haven't seen your bag; I don't know what you are talking about."

I calmly explained once again that I was told the protocol was that the bags were placed on shelves with our name tags on them and were brought up by porters after surgery.

She got a really angry look on her face. "I didn't steal your bag, Andrea; do you think I stole your bag? Why would I take your bag?"

I was flabbergasted; this nurse was completely nuts. I answered loudly now, as clearly no one was sleeping in this room with this crazy woman. "No I *don't* think you *stole* my bag. Have you even *looked* for it?"

Crossly, and with much indignation, she left. I waited for my toast. I waited and I waited and I waited. I was so desperate for it that I started drooling. Finally, my bed partner moved and grunted.

"What time is it?" I squeaked.

"Eleven thirty," he moaned. An hour so far, waiting for toast. I had to pee. Weakly, with my head spinning, I managed to get into an upright position. I nervously readied my legs, preparing to stand. I wore no underwear and for some reason my hospital johnnie shirt was ripped open at the shoulder and I had no robe. I wondered what had happened in the O.R. for the shoulder to be ripped open and my robe missing. With much wobbling and shuffling, I got myself to the bathroom. Although I knew better, I was in bare feet on the dirty hospital floors as my slippers were in the missing bag. The floor was filthy with urine and bits of toilet paper. I clumsily stepped in it with my bare feet as I was super dizzy from the drugs and weak from no food. My situation was simply miserable and should never have played out like this. I felt hugely frustrated by the treatment from the nurse and how long I was still waiting for the basics. Ultimately, I lost my patience. *Fuck this*, I thought to myself. I was angry. *Really* angry. I decided to force myself to walk down the hall. I was going to find this nurse and get that piece of toast.

I staggered out of the bathroom and, arms flailing, quickly grabbed onto the wide wooden rails on the wall. I took a deep breath. With eyes closed, I gritted my teeth and readied myself. *I'm doing this.* I pulled open the large hospital room door and stepped out into the bright light of the hall.

I squinted and felt dizzy again. With one arm I pushed the IV pole along with its tangled and numerous tubes; with the other I clutched the wooden railing and inched my way down the hall. The back of my johnnie shirt hung wide open and my pale butt brightly presented itself for all to see. I was well aware of this and yet didn't have a free hand to hold myself closed. I was so desperate, I made the choice to just be exposed. Down the long hallway I could see the nurses' station. Nurse Evil sat there at the computer. She didn't see me. I glared at her, as I slowly pulled myself along, ready for battle. Grunting, sweating, tears pouring down my face, I finally made it to the nurses' station. Nurse Evil finally looked up and appeared a little shocked to see me standing there, panting, hunched over in pain and covered in sweat.

It was indeed dangerous to be up and walking so far that soon after the surgery. Weak from no food, dizzy from the heavy meds, and unaccompanied, I was at great risk of falling down and could've really hurt myself. The effort it took to arrive at the desk was painful, and the bare butt exposure was humiliating. It was unthinkable that I needed to go through that. Nurse Evil regained her composure from my surprise arrival and looked straight at me, the teeniest of enjoyment registering in her eyes.

"Where's my TOAST?" I bellowed. The other two nurses quickly looked up from their work, and I could see by their faces they felt instantly upset on my behalf. Nurse Evil, totally put out, snapped back, "I was busy, Andrea. You're not the only one on this floor, you know."

The other nurses nervously glanced at each other. Their exchange said it all. *This nurse is terrible; we hate working with her.*

I looked back at Nurse Evil and could see her looking at something across the hallway. I followed her gaze, and to my ultimate shock, saw my bag. Right there. Ten feet across the hall in direct view from the nurses' station. I ambled over and realized this was a designated room for patients' bags. The nurses were to go to this room when the patient arrived and bring their overnight bag. Mine was the only one in there. It was obvious that my nurse knew it was there and had refused to bring it to me.

"My BAG!" I roared. Enough was enough. I was ready for combat. Let's GO! WWF in a cage. My eyes glazed over. I felt pure *rage*. Sweaty hair stuck to my face and teeth bared, ever so slowly I turned around and glowered at Nurse Evil. My chest heaved with effort and emotions; I was seething mad;

my rage, profound. Feeling my colossal wrath, she quietly got up and slunk down the hallway. I looked at the other two nurses who stood there, speechless and very upset, and I started crying all over again.

When you have a full hysterectomy, you cannot lift anything heavier than five pounds for the first eight weeks. It is extremely important to follow this rule, as otherwise you can destroy the inner stitches and have an internal bleed, or worse.

I looked at the remaining two nurses. Still shaking with both rage and utter weakness, I heard my voice falter. "Can one of you please carry my bag down to my room?"

A tall, beautiful, Amazonian braided beauty hopped up right away. She came over to me. I was so grateful and exhausted, tears streamed down my face. I looked up into her big kind eyes and simply asked, "Can I please hug you?"

She grinned a huge, bright, toothy grin and wrapped massive, strong arms around me that could've stretched all the way around an ancient California Redwood. I cried and hugged her as hard as I could. It was quite clear that I was traumatized. She patted me on the back and got me safely down the hall. I returned to my room with newfound coping skills as I dug in my bag for my slippers, some lip balm and some fresh underwear. I realized there was no way I could bend to get them on, as I had five puncture holes in my abdomen and was heavily stitched. This was, after all, major surgery.

Just then, Nurse Evil came in with the toast. I almost laughed, it was so incredibly ridiculous. Two hours of waiting for it when she knew I was weak and hungry. She stood there staring at me as I struggled to sit up. She handed me the paper plate with one cold, dry piece of whole wheat toast. "You'll have to put the peanut butter on it yourself," she spat. I was not sure how I would manage that with the IV in my dominant hand. I had fluid buildup and my hand looked like it belonged to the Pillsbury Doughboy. I couldn't hold the plastic knife and I couldn't get the peanut butter package open; Nurse Evil stood there, watching me struggle. Finally, I looked up at her.

"Hurry up!" she said. "Your toast is getting cold."

Through clenched teeth I said, "You're going to have to help me."

She looked at me. "Andrea, hysterectomy patients have to do things by themselves. You have to be ready to go home in the morning." And she promptly left.

I worked and worked at the peanut butter and finally got it open and on the toast. I chewed and chewed and chewed, and for the life of me could not get enough spit to swallow the damn bread. I reached for my bag and carefully dug around in the dark for a water bottle, trying not to further irritate the IV in my hand. All of a sudden, burning acid came rising up from my stomach and seared my throat. Instant esophageal pain. I was taken aback by the immediate agony of it. I tried to drink my water to no avail. I grabbed for my buzzer and pressed the blue button. Nothing. No response. I knew it was only a matter of seconds before I would be in further agony, and I knew it was unlikely my nurse was going to answer. I held down the button for a good ten seconds. "What?" I heard her answer, in complete exasperation.

"I need help," I squeaked.

After what seemed like forever, she arrived.

"I need some Gas-x or Tums or something."

She actually looked quite pleased. "See, Andrea? I told you, you should have waited until the morning before eating."

I begged her to get me something for the acid. She said "I cannot get you anything. It is not in your file from your doctor that you are to have this." She left abruptly again.

Holy fucking hell! I thought. *Am I in a movie? Is this actually happening?* I got up from bed again and for a second, painful time, I staggered out with my IV pole, again sweating profusely, hunched over in pain, taking one baby step after another. I walked down the long hallway, trying not to pass out. It took a tremendous amount of effort.

Thankfully, Amazon Queen was at the front desk this time. "I need help." I explained as politely and as calmly as I could, "I have severe heartburn." I looked so pathetic that I actually felt embarrassed. I was truly helpless. Without a word of debate, Amazon Queen got up, walked around the corner, and brought out a paper cup of liquid chalk. I hastily drank it down and tearfully thanked her.

And now, ever so slowly, I could feel the pain coming back from the surgery. I glanced at the nurses' station clock: two a.m. I was due for more narcotics. I dreaded the fact that I was going to have another interaction with my hateful nurse. I inched slowly back to my room. I assumed the nurses had times noted on their patients and would show up at the designated times to give the medicines. So I chose not to ring the buzzer. Sadly, that wasn't the case here on the sixth floor.

I waited in severe pain for another fifteen minutes and finally couldn't take a minute more. At 2:15 I again buzzed my nurse. This was an ongoing nightmare that just would not stop.

"What now, Andrea?" Nurse Evil was back at the desk intercom with more impatience.

"I need my meds."

"You just had your meds."

"No," I sighed, "I had them at ten p.m. It is now after two a.m. I am due for my meds."

"Do you think we just stare at the clock for you?"

I could not understand why she continued to twist every single thing I said. *Truly, this is manipulative, patient abuse at its finest.* After countless minutes, she came back with my meds. I was still trying to get slippers and underwear on by myself and so in need of sleep I felt delirious.

I dreaded asking her for help. "I need to get my underwear on. I cannot bend. Can you please assist me?"

"You want ME to help you get your underwear on?" She sounded indignant and truly annoyed. I thought to myself, *what the hell do you actually do as a nurse? Why is this so mind-blowing to you?*

With the severe pain, the constant mistreatment, and hours of trying to be patient, I burst out in long, loud moans. I was shocked at what I was hearing first from her, and then from me. I couldn't hold back my emotions any longer. More long, loud moans came from deep within my chest, like a wailing siren, followed by wracking, full-bodied sobs. I was aware of the scene I was now causing with my uncontrollable grief.

"Shh!" she hissed. "You are so inconsiderate of the other patients in here, Andrea."

I snapped my head around and I swear I saw red. Again seething at her, I officially lost it. "What is your name?" I roared. "What. Is. Your. Name? I am reporting you. You are going to be FIRED!" My entire body shook.

She smirked at me. "My name is Shelagh. You can't fire me."

"You should not be working here. You are awful to your patients." I was so angry in that moment, I swear my blood was at a full, rolling boil. She left. I lay there for several minutes huffing, puffing, sniffing, and still shaking. I felt terrible. I thought about how all of this appeared to the others in the room. Through tears and more sniffs, I whispered into the darkness to my roommates. "I am soooo, so, so sorry to all of you for all of this."

Out of the dark I could hear the sounds of three different bodies shifting in their beds, and then soothing voices. "It's okay, Andrea. It's going to be okay."

16
HELP ME . . .

I had had enough. I was deeply, intensely exhausted, and well beyond upset. I felt scared, vulnerable, abused, and completely shocked that this nurse was treating me this way. It was the first impression I had of how present-day in-patients were treated in hospital, and I silently prayed this nurse did not represent the majority of nurses. I was in need of a shower and I desperately wanted my family to come rescue me. I decided to text Mike to see if I could somehow, magically, be snuck out of the hospital. You know the scene: he sneaks in wearing a blue janitor's outfit, pushing a giant white laundry bin on wheels, sneaks into my room, meets me silently, and quick as a bunny I hop in to the bin and dive under all the laundry and out we go into the free world! It would be perfectly foolproof. If only I could put my hands on a janitor's outfit . . . . It was three a.m. and I decided to text him to see if he was awake.

Yo . . . You awake?

There she is. Hi, Wifey.

You need to come get me . . . NOW.

Hun?

This place is awful.

Well of course it is, it's a hospital . . .

*No, you don't understand, my nurse is
completely crazy.*

Really?

Yes. I am DEAD serious.

What's going on?

*She's actually yelled at me several times, she's
incredibly impatient, completely neglectful, and
just . . . awful. I can't stop crying. She is scaring me
and she continues to be late on my pain meds. I
ended up yelling back at her and told her she should
be fired. I'm in so much pain . . . I just need to
go home.*

Do you need me to come in?

*Yes, PLEASE!!!!!!!! I know you can't right now
though. OMGosh I'm so miserable, and exhausted.*

Try to get some sleep.

How early in the morning can you come????

What time would you like?

Like . . . 7 am.

*Ok, well I have to deal with walking and feeding
Duey, and then driving all the way in, so it might be
later than that. Try and rest. You'll be ok. I love you.*

Ok I'll try. I love you too so much. Please hurry.

17
THE NEXT DAY

"Yay! Blood lady! Blood lady is here!"

I woke up to a singsong Asian voice. It was only just a few short hours after I had texted Mike in the middle of the night to come rescue me. It took me a moment before I opened my eyes. A teeny, energetic, smiling young woman squeezed into the curtains alongside the bed of the woman across from me. "Hello. Good morning!" she sang.

"Good morning!" the woman across from me said back to her. They both sounded quite pleasant.

"How are you do-ing to-day?" She was full-out singing.

The patient laughed. "Oh, not too badly."

Moments later I heard "All done!" and she promptly moved to the other bed on that side, another lady. This was my first glance at the two women who had heard all of the commotion and upset last night. I watched in awe as the "blood lady" collected blood efficiently and effortlessly.

She crossed over to the man next to me. "Hey, Ray!" She smiled brightly at him. "How's Ray today?"

"Ray's good!" Ray said. He turned to look at me and his eyes widened. I had managed to put some makeup on. I am sure they were all picturing an absolute hag of a madwoman, instead of me sitting there, youthful, fresh-faced, and with long, auburn, French braids. I had chosen braids to keep my hair out of the way in surgery, and they were still neatly doing their job. Ray's smile told me he was in a great deal of pain, but at least he was smiling. "This lady here, she's real slick," he said, nodding at the blood tech. I smiled back. *We will see about that when she reaches my stupid veins*, I wanted to reply.

Seconds later, she came to my side of the bed. It was a tight squeeze for her; this room was only a double and yet four large beds were crowded in here.

"Hi, pretty girl." she said. "You have favourite arm?"

I smiled at her. She sure lit up the room. "No, I have challenging veins. They roll, they're tiny, and very deep."

"No problem! That's 'cause you are warrior. You keep veins safe." I liked her thinking. I took a deep breath. She stood there, not touching my arms at all. "I have selected one! You ready for me?"

I was confused. *How could I be ready? Had she even found a good vein?* She hadn't picked up either arm, hadn't tapped away with her two fingers, no tourniquet.

"Uh, okay, yup," I stammered. I was so tired; I'd had only four hours of sleep.

"In we go . . . and . . . we're all done!"

What? How was that possible? Was she joking? I looked around and saw her holding up a vial of dark purple blood. I had not felt a thing. *How did she do that?* I looked at her face. She was smiling big smiles.

"Okay! Blood lady says, bye-bye! You rest now, pretty lady." And just like that, she was gone. I turned to look at Ray. He was laughing, almost.

"What did I tell ya?" he said. "She's the best I've ever had."

I looked at the clock: 7:20. Still exhausted, I closed my eyes tight to block out the morning sunlight and promptly fell asleep.

I was in a small, warm, circular pool of water. There were several pools all around, but I was alone, gently swishing my arms back and forth in green murkiness in which I was fully immersed. I could hear water running behind me, a soft, gentle trickle landing in a pool below, like a small waterfall. It was dark; stars shone overhead and mist rose up from the pools. It was a dimly lit area and I could just see the moonlight through a few trees; there was dangling foliage hanging all around me. The air was heavy, moist.

All of a sudden, there was a beautiful, young sorceress sitting across from me in the water. How had she entered without my knowledge? She looked friendly, so I smiled. She had long black hair that seductively wound around her arms and breasts and her green, mesmerizing eyes shone; cat-like. She sat quietly staring at me. After a few minutes, her elongated arms stretched toward me. I was just out of reach. She leaned her head and torso in closer to me and reached again.

I didn't like what she was doing, and I discreetly edged closer to the back of the pool, but the edge was no longer there. It had disappeared and now behind me I could feel thick, cold gel preventing me from gently moving away. She was still reaching for me, and I saw that her fingernails were several inches long. The ends curled into spirals, painted bright silver with gold jewels encrusting them. Gilded rings were on every finger, and her arms were wound with many gold bracelets dangling under a sleeve of fine fabric that had been cut into long, large triangles. Somehow I knew that the robes went all the way to her feet. They were a soft blue and made of expensive silk. She opened her heavily painted lips.

"Andreahh," she whispered to me, drawing out my name. My brows furrowed—I was surprised she knew my name—and her eyes became slits. Her lips slowly curled into a small, mysterious smile. Her robes stayed dry even though she was fully immersed in the warm murkiness that now was turning a darker, colder green. She stood up and I watched the water droplets fall off of her dry robes. Suddenly her gown turned into ripped, dirty rags. "Andreahhh," she whispered again, drawing out my name even longer, and I looked up and saw that this time grey smoke was pouring from her mouth. It rose up into the air, swirling, and remained just above her head. I looked back to her face and suddenly I felt sick with dread. She smiled at me again and I watched in fear as her tongue turned into that of a serpent's, long and black; it split in two and kept flicking at me, getting longer and longer. "Andreaaaaahhh." Her voice had changed from a whisper to a loud, crackling moan.

She was so close now, I could smell her breath. It smelled as though something was rotting deep inside her. I started to make a large move to get away, but when I looked into her eyes I froze in terror; they had turned a glowing, fiery red. My heart pounded. Smoke poured out from her mouth again and she rose up high from the water, towering well above my head. She looked about fifteen feet tall as she glided toward me. With one swift swish of my arms, I somehow managed to get about fifteen feet away from her. I tried to scream but my voice wouldn't come out—

"Andrea! Wake up!"

My eyes flew open. A nurse was there, checking my temp and stats. The heavy narcotics in me were messing with my REM sleep, big time. I was confused, having been awoken from such heavy sleep, but I was relieved to see that I was back in the hospital—it was better than being in the murky green pool with the sorceress.

I dozed in and out as early morning wore on. I would fall asleep and then awaken over and over again. Someone would come in, a breakfast delivery would get dropped off, a nurse would check on one of us, a noisy IV alarm would need attention, a visitor would drop by for one of the other patients— I was amazed at how little sleep one gets in the hospital and quickly realized, a hospital is no place for the sick.

Mike arrived at about eight thirty and to say I was totally overjoyed to see him was an understatement. He'd come for a quick check-in before heading to work and could tell I'd barely slept. I was totally overwhelmed and for that he looked concerned about me. We assumed I'd be discharged that morning as protocol dictated, but we didn't yet know when. While he was in there we met the day nurse. She was bubbly and sweet and had a skip to her sneakered step. Nurse Evil had finished her shift and I was quite relieved about that; I could feel my body finally relax a little bit. After a few more minutes I told Mike and the nurse that I wanted to try to rest, and so Mike left for work. I again dozed in and out, feeling like I could sleep for years.

"Hi, Andrea!" Another perky voice. I opened my eyes and saw my angel, Dr. Scott, standing next to my bed with her white coat and stethoscope. She was so darn kind—it exuded from her pores. I was so glad to see her that I forgot about my surgery and tried to sit upright a little too fast. Instantly I felt a heavy pain in my left side, and I winced. "Just stay put, my dear." She placed hands on my legs and looked at me, almost amused that I was so excited to see her.

"How's the pain overall?"

"Manageable."

"Have you peed?"

"Yes."

"Have you been up out of the room yet?"

A flashback to me baring my teeth at Nurse Evil and yelling loudly about my bag. "Uh, yes."

"Okay, great. I think you will be discharged today."

"Oh Yay!" I cheered with relief. And then I looked at Ray and the others. "I mean, it's not that I don't like you people—you're great. I'm just really ready to go home!"

They chuckled. "Don't worry, we understand."

I turned to Dr. Scott. "What do you make of my chest pain?" I asked. I had told Nurse Evil last night that my chest had been paining a lot, but she hadn't really checked anything. Dr. Scott looked down at me now, a little more serious.

"You have chest pain?" she asked.

"Yes. It started last night. *Likely the stress from Shelagh.*

Dr. Scott did some assessments—pressing, listening, asking more questions. After a few moments she said, "Well, I don't like that. We are going to have to get you in for a CT scan just to rule out any blood clots. I don't feel comfortable sending you all the way out to Peggy's Cove. It doesn't make sense to risk anything when we can check this out while you're here. It might take a while to get you in—are you okay with that?"

How could I say no? "Okay. Yup. Thank you." I smiled.

Immediately I worried that Shelagh would be back on again while I was still in hospital, and I laid there feeling nervous and overtired. My johnnie shirt was pulled way up over my belly, exposing my sutures; they were driving me crazy, so very sore and now for some reason quite itchy, and I couldn't stand the feel of anything touching them. Dr. Scott surveyed me lying there, feeling vulnerable and mildly irritated. "Can I get you anything?" I was so amazed by her. Imagine, a surgeon asking me this. Mind-blowing.

"Yes, you can actually. Can you drive to my house and bring my two-hundred-pound mastiff back to cheer me up?"

She chuckled and I saw a twinkle in her eye as she left.

At this point Ray started talking to me, and he politely asked if he could pull back the curtain. "Sure." I replied, although in truth I wanted to close my eyes and get back to the restorative rest I so desperately needed. Wrinkled, arthritic, yellowed hands came around to my side of the curtain, and he pulled it so that we could lie there talking face to face. We were really crammed in there, our beds so close that we looked like husband and wife having a bedtime chat.

"Hi." He smiled.

"Well hello there, handsome." I smiled back. I was trying hard to bring a cheer to his heart. He was not actually handsome in a typical way. He was weathered, unwell, and had very little energy left in him. He had messy, dirty blond hair, a tanned face, blue eyes that I bet once sparkled, and deep lines in his face. Before his illness he was likely a decent-looking man, but you could tell he likely smoked all his life and had had a rough go; it took away from some of those nice features.

"Are you Dutch?" I asked. He had the depth of a Dutchman. He seemed grounded and confident, warm and friendly.

"What gave it away?" He smiled at me, intrigued.

"I just know a few Dutch people. I love them." I'd actually been engaged to a Dutchman years and years before. He was tall, handsome, with blue eyes and a smile to die for. He had an amazing family with six siblings: one brother and five sisters. I didn't marry him—our paths were misaligned—but I was left with a long-lasting impression of Dutch men and could spot one instantly.

Ray and I ended up chatting for several hours, and he told me he was dying. He had cancer in many parts of his body and would not be leaving the hospital. He was clearly in pain and needed a lot of drugs to keep him comfortable. I shared with him the many challenges of my life and my out-look on them, and he just kept looking at me and saying, "You are remark-able. You have such a positive attitude!"

His words surprised me. "Well you kinda have to, right?" I replied, feel-ing emotional and proud at the same time. I told him I was a big optimist. "Happiness is a choice," I reasoned. "I come away from the more challenging situations asking myself what was the lesson, what did I gain, and how could I do better. I try to treat others with kindness and I try to leave people in a brighter mood than when I first met them, although . . ." I paused for a moment thinking about the interactions with Nurse Evil, "you wouldn't have that impression of me after last night." I was embarrassed, but the other patients all seemed not to worry about it, as if they knew Shelagh was like that with everyone.

"Remarkable," he said again, looking at me. After a while we both started drifting off.

"Okay, Ray, time for your scan." We both woke with a start. A porter had shown up, speaking loudly. They wheeled Ray away. I felt a sadness to see him go, as I didn't know if I would ever see him again. It's like that in hospitals—you never know when something is going to happen or what comes next.

Mike texted a check-in at lunchtime and I told him I was not going home yet but that I was really hungry and not able to eat much of the hospital food. He showed up in the early afternoon with a cheeseburger. Never in my life have I been happier to eat one; I gobbled it down in three bites. My stomach did not enjoy it as much as my mouth did however, and it protested in loud, high-pitched squeaking sounds not unlike the air being squeezed from an overfilled balloon. I was relieved to see him again; we finally got to talk in person instead of texts. In whispers, I told him all about the horrible night with Nurse Evil. He looked deeply concerned and annoyed. Just then the cheery nurse from the morning visit came back; she was accompanied by a male nurse and they talked to us for a bit. It felt a little like old friends had come to visit. She gave me more pain meds and told Mike the plan for my chest scan. I asked them how the nurses' shifts worked, and then Mike realized what I was actually trying to ask, and so he asked more directly if I would have the same nurse that night as I had the night before. I held my breath in fear. "Yes, that's how it works," they replied, not so enthusiastically.

I burst into tears and started to shake. There was no way I could manage another night with Nurse Evil. The three of them looked at me, upset and worried. I was experiencing tremendous anxiety over how I had been treated the night before, my body providing proof of my strong feelings, my inability to cope, and just how truly bad the experience was.

Mike immediately came to my defence. "Look." he said, his face full of concern. "My wife gets along with everybody. *Literally* everybody. If she's reacting like this, then I know it's been bad. This is not like her at all." He paused for a moment and then added, "There is no way she's going to have that nurse again, and if I have to sleep on this bed tonight to make sure she's okay, I will do just that." *Go Mike!* I thought, smiling to myself. I was so impressed. I love how my husband always has my back.

The two nurses looked at each other. It was quite obvious they knew about this nurse.

"By the looks on your faces, this is no surprise to either of you, and I bet you know exactly who we're talking about." More directness from Mike.

They quietly whispered that I was not the first person to have a complaint about her. They said they would speak to their supervisor and would try to get a different nurse for me. This was helpful and I felt somewhat relieved. Mike stayed a while longer and I finally felt safe, knowing he was there. Eventually, I started to fall asleep again.

I woke up when Ray came back. He was in a tremendous amount of pain and had a hard time transferring back to his bed from the stretcher. He buzzed for a nurse and asked for pain management. Nurse Evil walked in. "What, Ray?"

My stomach dropped. *She was back!* My heart started pounding and I averted my eyes.

"Hi there," Ray said calmly to her. "Could I possibly have some pain meds? I am in a great deal of pain right now."

She sighed loudly like he'd just asked her to drag an elephant in to saddle up. "Just a minute," she snapped, spinning on her heel as she left.

I was confused. *I thought she was going to be switched out of here?* Then it dawned on me that maybe it was only for *me* that she was switched, but I would still have to see her coming in and out as there were three other patients in the room. To hear her treating the others so poorly made me very unhappy—powerless and scared. I felt like I was back in grade school, dealing with a bully.

When I was in grade nine, there was a girl who was really jealous of me because her boyfriend had a wee crush. He would greet me each day as I got off the school bus and would cheerily carry my trombone up to the band room for me. I was grateful, as the instrument was quite heavy. I thought it odd that he would be so brazen while dating her, but I happily accepted the help, naively assuming that she was okay with him doing that. Well, guess what? She was not, at all. This went on for months and she glared at me in the hallways like she wanted to tear my limbs off and stick them up my nose, or perhaps even worse places. She started threatening to beat me up, and I went to school each day terrified of her. It culminated in her cornering me in the bathroom during our grade nine prom at the end of June. She smacked me hard across the face, leaving a pink hand mark. She ruined my prom and once again I had trembling fingers in a rotary phone calling my dad to the rescue.

The same feelings of dread, fear, and anxiety were coming up now with Shelagh still in my world. I was angry that she had treated Ray like this, yet I was afraid to speak up. In such a weakened state, I felt vulnerable, powerless. She came back and gave Ray some pills to swallow. "Thank you very much," Ray said with a smile.

After he got settled, he and I resumed talking and shared each other's cancer journeys. "What?" he said in surprise. "*You* had cancer? I thought you were just in for a routine hysterectomy." I told him the whole story of how I was so unwell and irregularly symptomatic and how my GP had basically missed the entire thing. He was amazed. "That's just awful," he said. "I am so sorry." Ray and I talked for several more hours and I came to really care for him.

The afternoon slowly moved into dinner time, and we ate the hospital food trying to make light of the mysterious things under the plate cover. I did end up having a different nurse, who was attentive, polite, and quick with my meds. I still didn't like the heavy pain in my chest and lower left side. My stitches were really making me itchy, and I kept going from hot and sweaty to cold and shivery. "You have a fever," my kind nurse said as she waited for the beep of the thermometer. She was right. I was surprised and a little concerned as I rarely get fevers. It was not super high, mind you, but still not a comfortable situation after major surgery.

I tried to sleep a little more, and at about eleven o'clock two paramedics came in and woke me. "Andrea?" I opened my eyes to see them standing there, almost against the wall, with virtually no room to move. "We're here to take you over to the other hospital for your CT." I was confused. *This hospital doesn't have a machine?* "We have to get you ready for ambulance transport." I took in their chiseled, manly faces. *Oh, this might be fun.* I thought, desperate to get out of there. I had only been in an ambulance once before, when I was five.

Thinking back to that experience, I recalled we had just arrived in New Brunswick; another one of our Winter break trips to visit our Nana, and Mom had sent us out to play. We badly needed some fresh air and Mom likely needed a strong cup of tea after another long car ride. I had my favorite shiny purple snow suit on and I felt like a superhero in it.

In the back of Nana's house there was a long, sloping hill that I was itching to slide down. "Do you have any crazy carpets Nana?" I'd asked, joyfully. "No dear, I don't, I'm sorry." Disappointed, I thought for a moment. "A black garbage bag perhaps?" She looked curiously at me. "What are you going to do with that?" she'd inquired. "I'm going to use it to slide down the hill!" I explained excitedly, grinning my toothless grin. "Well alright dear, they're kept in the pantry closet." So off I went, grabbing a bag and getting outside before you could even say "Bob's your Uncle."

It was cold out and the hill was covered in ice from the Maritime weather alternating between heavy snow and freezing rain. I sat down on the garbage bag, and then carefully laid down on my back, grabbing my feet and hoisting them high in the air; like an upside down turtle. I wriggled and inched my butt along to get going, grunting as I went. Lara was happily trying to build a snowman with recently fallen snow just below the roof of the house. There, the snow was still damp and heavy instead of crusted and hard-packed. "What are you doing?" she asked nervously. "C'mon! Slide down the hill with me!" I replied with excitement. She looked at the long, steep, icy hill that had a five foot drop off at the bottom over a rock wall into the neighbor's place below. "Are you crazy?" she asked. I looked back at her. *Why would she ask that?* "It looks a-maz-ing!" I yelled, I was starting to feel impatient.

She continued to work on her snowman as I grunted my way along to the top of the hill, where it dropped down at a very steep angle. As an adult with years of experience down-hill skiing, I would say that that hill had a pretty steep pitch. So yes; I was indeed crazy. At the time though, for some reason, it looked fun. "Wheeeeeee!" I yelled as I finally got going. Hard packed ice bumps lifted me up off the hill and landed me with thump after hard thump numerous times as I went. "Ooof-ow-ow-whoa-oof-oof-yow!" I screeched as I flew along, quickly approaching the rock wall at the end. My heart pounded. "Wheeeeeee!!" I screeched again as I was lifted higher off the ground. I flew through the air at maximum speed, and then . . . falling . . . falling and landing hard on the ice below. "Oomph" my body made an abnormal sound as the wind got knocked out of me. I continued to speed along even with the hard landing. I dug my boots into the snow as hard as I could, applying the brakes as I rapidly approached a large tree. Cold snow pushed up the legs of my snow suit and filled the top of my boots. My exposed skin burned from the icy bits that scraped me and I gasped for air as I came to a grinding halt at the base of a tree. "That was stupendous!" I screeched even louder, breathlessly yelling to my sister.

And then began the long ascension up the hill. Icy breath came out of me as I huffed and panted along. Crunch-crunch-crunch, my boots caved through the crispy snow as I moved. I reached the rock wall and saw a little tree next to it. *I'd really like to climb that tree!* I checked out the prospects. It was a young tree without many low branches to put my feet on. I reached up and grabbed for a limb overhead and saw that it was just out of reach. I jumped up and down several times, wondering why my super-hero snowsuit was failing me.

"Lara!" I called loudly. "Come lift me up!" I pictured her bending over with her hands out so that I could just step into them and she could hoist. "No Andrea! You'll hurt the tree. It's a baby and not strong enough!" she called back. I begged her. She refused. My sister has been a tree lover her whole life and there was no way she was going to risk snapping a limb on this little one.

"Idea!" I said out loud as I put my wet mittened hand on my chin. I assessed the rock wall in front of me. *If I climbed up onto the top of the wall, I could launch myself into the tree limb and then climb the rest.* I crunched over to the wall. I put my foot into an opening, and began to wiggle and climb. Unexpectedly, rocks loosened, and the wall came down on top of me. "Ow!" I cried out, as I laid on my back in the snow. What I had thought were rocks were actually big, loose, heavy construction blocks. I felt a dull pain in my lower left leg and laid there for a few moments trying to catch my breath. The sun was shining brightly down on me but I was getting cold. I used my right leg to try to push the block off as it was on an angle over my left leg. I couldn't do it. "Lara!" I called. I didn't know if she could actually see me as I was on the other side of the wall, but I quickly realized I was stuck and needed someone to get down that icy hill to help me. "Lara!!" I called louder. Slowly I started to panic. I'd really hurt myself. "I need help!" I cried out. She, of course, thought I was faking. We used to do this kind of stuff all of the time, as siblings do. A few more moments passed. "Lara!!" I screamed louder still. "I'm serious. Help me!"

She carefully inched down the steep, icy hill and saw me laying there, the mess of blocks all around me. Quickly she jumped off the wall and raced over, trying to get the block off my leg. "I'm going to get Mom!" she said breathlessly, as she took in the whole situation. I watched as she turned around and slipped and slid her way back up the icy hill, her feet continually sliding out from under her. We had been at Nanas for less than ten minutes. My poor mother had not even taken her own shoes off, and to my surprise and wonderment saw her race out in high heels, blouse and a skirt; she hadn't even grabbed her winter coat. She dug her heels into the ice and carefully picked her way down the steep hill until she stood over me.

Quickly she got the concrete block off and assessed the situation. I actually don't remember being in a great deal of pain. Perhaps I was in shock, or perhaps it was so cold in the snow that I'd lost feeling, but I remember telling her that I could not feel my leg. She yelled back up the hill to Lara. "Go tell Nana to call an ambulance!"

Mom stayed there with me, and sure enough an ambulance came a short while later. She shivered, likely regretting not grabbing a coat but in typical mother fashion, reacted as fast as she could, to help her child.

The paramedics assessed me and told Mom my leg was likely broken. I remember a big strong man carrying me back up the hill in his arms and I felt like a small animal hitching a ride on its' father; my busy mind working overtime. Ultimately the other paramedic was at the top of the hill, waiting with the stretcher. They loaded me in and Mom rode with me to the hospital in the back of the ambulance. I shivered with the cold, and I think I may have peed in my snowsuit; it was quite soggy and heavy.

They prepped me for X-ray and I remember waking up to a full leg cast from hip to toe with just my little piggies sticking out. It was itchy and awful. I spent the whole Winter break in a cast, sitting on Nana's couch shoving metal clothes hangers down the inside of my cast to scratch my hot, itchy skin. At the end of our vacation I had to take a plane back to Halifax by myself as I couldn't make the drive home in the back seat of the car for five hours with the full leg cast. It was an expensive and harrowing week for us all.

"And lift on three." the paramedics said, as they raised me into the back of the ambulance, and I was abruptly brought back to my current situation. "In ya go." They bumped me around and I cried out in pain. This was followed by more bumps and more pain. They fastened the belts and I was grateful for the warm flannel blankets as it was a cold, frosty February night.

Big, fat, snowflakes flew all around. It was quite surreal, the three of us out at midnight, me getting loaded into an ambulance, the crisp air making me shiver and my teeth chatter. That ride was rough. Winter in Halifax means many potholes and the paramedics kept apologizing over and over for all of the bumps; every one they hit made me cry out.

Moaning and groaning and holding my abdomen, I reconsidered my enthusiasm for the ambulance. "Are you okay?" asked the young paramedic riding with me.

"No," I said, trying hard not to cry out as silent tears rolled down my face. "I just had a hysterectomy, and every pothole makes my insides feel like they are coming loose."

"Oh dear," he said. "This is an exceedingly bumpy, cold ride for someone freshly operated on. I am very sorry."

I was in agony when I got to the other hospital. They brought me to the scan room and two technicians were waiting for me. Fortunately, they were able to attach the dye needed into my already existing IV port, so all in all things went pretty smoothly. I was brought back to the other hospital again by the same paramedics and it was another miserable, bumpy ride. I felt like my innards were all shifting around and the stitches were getting destroyed. I was immensely relieved to climb back in bed, sometime well after midnight.

18
GOING HOME

The next morning, the singing, super-slick blood collection lady arrived again at seven o'clock sharp, and, just like the day before, drew my blood with no issues. I was amazed.

Various people came in and out that morning. Mom arrived for a quick visit and it was wonderful to see her smiling face. As intuitive as ever, she could tell that besides my surgery pain, something else was wrong. I didn't want to say too much about the blow out I'd had with Nurse Evil not that long ago, as I was worried she would want to march on out to the nurses' station and clout that awful Nurse Evil right in the nose.

I watched as she surveyed the room. She looked around at the dirty floors, drops of blood and tissues strewn about. Her face showed surprise as she took in the many containers, trays, Band-Aids, and discarded IV lines in the nearby sink. There was an outburst of sudden laughter and a cheer out in the hallway, and she shook her head at the noise. Taking a long breath in, her mouth formed a tight line of annoyance. "Nursing is certainly *not* what it used to be boy, I'll tell you that."

In Mom's nursing days, things were kept immaculate. Nurses wore pressed uniforms and their hair was kept up in a tight bun. They would never, EVER be rude to a patient, accuse them of wrongdoing, or belittle them like Nurse Evil had done to me. One would likely be fired on the spot if they'd acted like that.

Mom looked up as Ray squeezed past us to get to the bathroom. "Hello," he said. Mom smiled at him. "Is this your daughter?" he asked.

"Why yes, this is my pride and joy." Mom smiled back.

After a few moments, Ray came out and managed to get back into his bed even though he was in great pain and incredibly weak. Mom got up and went to his bedside.

"How are you doing? Do you need anything?" she asked. *God love Mama.*

"I'm okay, thank you. You look familiar. Are you a politician?" Ray asked, still sharp as a whip even with all of the pain meds.

Mom smiled and said, "That was one of my many careers, yes, but I'm also a former nurse. Can I be of any help?"

Ray smiled and thanked her. They started whispering and I strained to hear them, as I thought it odd they were whispering. "Your daughter is a giant ray of light. She's just remarkable. She has such a huge, positive attitude; I feel very encouraged by her. I'd given up, you know. They had the priest come in, but now, after talking to Andrea, I'm feeling a newfound lease on life. I have better mental health since she arrived. She's a wonderful young lady."

I was floored. I didn't know I had had that impact on him.

Mom, beaming, said, "Yes, Andrea has that effect on people."

A short while later I said goodbye to Mom and finally dozed a bit. I woke up to find Dr. Scott had come in to see me and she had good news—I was going home!

I called Mike, who was close by at his office. He arrived soon thereafter to collect my things and to take me home. With much thoughtfulness, he brought me a wheelchair as I was too weak to make the long walk to the car.

It was a stormy afternoon with high winds and ice pellets, and we drove with caution. It's one thing to drive through poor weather when you're in good health, a whole other when your insides have been removed and you've been sewn back together.

On our way, we made a stop at the house of one of my guitar students, Natalie. She had organized a food drive for me among my guitar ladies. I was lying in the SUV with the seat all the way down and I watched in awe as countless bag after bag of casseroles and muffins, cards, and gift baskets were loaded into the car. Tears filled my eyes as I took in the loving, kind efforts of it all. I was amazed at Natalie's kindness. She had not only orchestrated the huge food train, but had also coordinated pick-ups and drop-offs and had carefully stored it all as well. "Looks like your guitar ladies really love you," Mike said.

It is quite challenging for a cancer patient to go through a diagnosis and operation, and it's vitally important to have good support through it all. I was reminded again of how very fortunate I am to have such wonderful friends in my life; it helped a great deal when I was in such rough shape from the surgery and so weak from having had cancer. I certainly was not up to the task of making food and cleaning up, and Mike was swamped working full-time and looking after house chores and the dog. The thought of us having to manage groceries and cooking was daunting, and I was relieved to see the meals and baked goods.

As we continued to make our way, the weather became worse and worse; the temperature dropped and the winds increased, howling loudly. Mike did his best to avoid the bumps and holes in the road, and yet even still, I felt tremendous pain as we made our way; it brought me to silent tears over and over again, and I had difficulty coping. I was majorly sleep deprived, still somewhat traumatized, and my surgical wounds were quite raw.

When we finally arrived home, the house was unexpectedly very cold. I was truly desperate for a shower as I longed to get cleaned up and cozy but to my dismay, the strong winds had knocked the power out. With no running water, we also couldn't flush the toilets. Mike wanted to build a fire, but he knew that the strong north wind would likely cause the house to fill with smoke.

Now frozen, I painfully climbed into the bed in the guest room and Mike covered me from head to toe with a thick hat, a big sweater over my jammies, thick socks, and five heavy blankets. Bringing my hands out to eat a snack brought cold air to them, and I hurriedly ate and tucked them back under the covers. Mike was so cold he wore a hat, his fleece vest, a wool sweater, a ski jacket, and even his snow pants over long underwear and fleece pants. It was a ridiculous situation. As the miserable hours wore on, he asked me if I wanted to go over to the family cottage where there was a generator; we could have a bit of heat and some power. I was in so much pain from the ambulance the night before and then the long, bumpy ride home, I couldn't bear another second in a vehicle. Honestly, I swore if I got in a car again my stitches would let loose and I would bleed all over the seat.

By late afternoon the temperature had dropped to minus thirty outside and the strong northwest wind howled ferociously. Mike had to tape the windows shut to stop the powerful drafts coming directly off the ocean. We still had no power, and shockingly the house got down to a very chilly seven degrees Celsius. It was terrible conditions for someone freshly cut open and sewn back up. I tried hard not to take the prescribed morphine, but after a while the pain became unbearable. I ended up feverish and chilled and profusely sweating. Mike brought me several more blankets, water, and a sandwich and did his best to look after me while trying to manage the issues caused by the power outage. Ultimately we made it through the night.

The next morning, I woke up to my stitches irritating me even more than in the hospital. I had five big areas where I was stitched, and they were crusting and bleeding. Red, itchy splotches were all around the sutures and they began spreading into larger, more painful diameters. It was hard to look at them without feeling nauseated. I found out later that I was allergic to the material used to sew me up. Even with that extra bother, I was still feeling relieved to be home and glad I had gotten through it all.

By mid-morning the power had come back on and I was grateful that I once again had the use of heat and lights. TV, Sudoku puzzles, and video calls got me through the afternoon. I was told I could expect to be completely healed in about eight weeks. I wasn't allowed to drive a car until then, because if I were to have a fender-bender, I could bleed internally, so I was quite limited in what I could do.

Two days after getting home, I started to feel a little less awful, and I started walking slowly to the bathroom and kitchen. I missed my daughters; I needed to see them. A few days later, they showed up carrying a large pink basket. Their faces wore huge, excited smiles. I was immensely pleased and equally surprised to see that the two of them had put together incredibly thoughtful, and useful gifts—slippers, lip balm, hand cream, face masks, bubble bath, games, puzzles, colouring books, two little stuffed animals, and some tea. It had clearly taken quite a bit of time and money to put this all together.

"Oh my gosh, girls!" I said, teary with joy as I opened the delicately wrapped, tissue-papered surprises. "These gifts are just the best. How very kind and thoughtful of you to do this for me!"

Annie smiled and said, "Well we had a pretty good role model." and Maddie added, "You have taken such good care of us, now it's our turn to do something special for you!" and again I was amazed and proud of how mature they were.

Four days after the surgery, I posted an update to my friends, as people had started texting me to see about my status.

Social Media Post #2
February 5

I'm baaaaaack! ♡

I survived my surgery. (Holy hell, the pain). Peeps, I'm still on morphine and barely out of bed but just wanted to jump on here to say THANK YOU. I couldn't have gotten through this without you. Sincerely. The comments, prayers, check-ins, and love I received from you was what gave me strength, hope, and courage. The surgeon said things went well, and I look forward to getting the final results in a few weeks' time to hopefully be cancer-free. I'll update again then. In the meantime, just know that I'm eternally grateful for each and every one of you and very, very lucky.

Love ya!!

19

POOP, POOP-BA DOOP, POOP-BA DOOP, POOP-BA DOOPA-DOOPA-DOOP

As the days passed, I slowly settled into more routine. I re-read the "At Home Care" pamphlet and when I'd finished, reflected on the messages that really stood out from the whole hospital experience. I recalled that several nurses *heavily* reminded me that there was a risk of severe constipation after the surgery. This terrified me. I was amazed at just how many of the staff made it their top priority to communicate this. "Andrea, it's very, very important that you don't get constipated." "Andrea, do you have any Colace or RestoraLAX at home to take once you are discharged?" "Andrea, has anyone talked to you about the importance of staying well hydrated and eating fibre so that you don't have any issues when you get home?" "Have you been chewing your gum, Andrea, to stimulate your bowels?" and on and on and on it went. I have to admit; I was starting to get a little paranoid.

I knew quite well the colossal damage constipation can cause. I have been plagued with bowel issues for over twenty-five years and was certainly not wanting any part of that while still so deeply in pain from the operation itself. And, up until now, my bowel issues were really only known to me. I was hoping to keep it that way, but after reflecting upon what I went through, I felt compelled to share this experience, in the hope that you will come to really understand the true importance of not getting constipated. I promise, someday, you will thank me. And if you know someone who has been through the severe fecal impaction I am about to describe, they likely were too embarrassed to tell you the worst of the horrific details. Go and hug them just the same and tell them you now have a much better understanding of what they went through. Furthermore, for the people who *have* been through this, know that you are not alone and that you are incredibly resilient to still be walking upright! Ah, yes. We can joke about it now, but I am being quite serious. The months it took for this incident to heal left me wondering if I would ever be able to sit, stand, walk, or dance ever again. I'm not kidding. And now a wee tribute to my other dear grandmother, as she clearly was ahead of her time with preventative measures back in the late '70s.

Grammy would make the long journey from New Brunswick to our Bedford home and would always bring a can of prune juice with her for the duration of her stay, usually about a week. Lara and I would sneak down to the kitchen, peer into the refrigerator, and look at the giant can of prune juice somewhat hidden on the bottom shelf. Lara would start giggling and whisper to me, "Andrea, what's that prune juice for?" and I would devilishly whisper back, "To make Grammy pooooop!" and we would burst into absolute fits of laughter while trying our best to be quiet. Well. I should've taken Grammy's lead on that one and bought some damn prune juice.

Even with much experience in this department, I still didn't fully understand just how dangerous *severe* constipation could actually get, even with those nurses looking at me so sternly. In hindsight I guess they couldn't exactly say, "Andrea, I don't mean to scare you, but you will be in horrifyingly unbearable pain if you let this situation get out of hand."

I have often wondered how I would've fared if only I'd taken an entire *cup* of RestoraLAX and not just a capful, perhaps *ten* Colace pills and not just two, and maybe *the entire freaking box* of ex-lax. Maybe, just maybe, I wouldn't have experienced that horrible, fateful day.

Because I'm fair-skinned and red-haired, my skin and nerve endings are much more tender than the average person, and I can confidently say that it has been well documented by surgeons and dentists alike that red-haired people require a lot more sedation and pain meds to manage surgeries and procedures than all other types of people. So when I even have occasional *mild* constipation issues at home, sadly, they are *excruciating.*

During my surgery, I was given something to induce gastro paresis or, to clarify, to paralyze the bowels so that they wouldn't move during surgery. Why? Because if a bowel gets nicked by a surgeon's knife (or in this case a robotic one), it could potentially cause the perforated bowel to slowly leak into the rest of the body, which can be fatal. Surgeons also want to avoid a patient's spontaneous bowel movement, as an unexpected movement can be tricky while operating and an unexpected evacuation can allow bacteria to spread. Besides, who wants a patient to poop while you're operating on them?

Post-op, I was given a stool softener so that I would not get constipated. When you are warned there is a danger of severe constipation, you take your medicine. I did so, faithfully. I drank RestoraLAX twice a day to get things really soft, and . . . nothing. I also drank a ton of water and ate fibrous foods, and yet . . . still nothing. I could hear my stomach gurgling at various times throughout the day, and I was getting more and more bloated as time wore on. I would feel like I had to go, and then, I would sit, wait, and . . . nothing would happen. I felt heavy and bloated as the contents of my bowels were completely stuck, deep inside me. I didn't know what else to do, so I kept throwing things at it, silently praying I wouldn't spontaneously combust. I remained constipated. Severely, horribly, painfully, and humiliatingly constipated.

My mind kept nervously returning to my grade five science project, the erupting volcano with thick brown lava bubbling and exploding out of the hole, and I regularly implored a silent request that that wouldn't be me once it all decided to let loose. I even imagined a balloon that had not been tied off and was let go, flying all around the room, making a high-pitched squeal. *What if I produce so much gas I start flying all around the room, making high-pitched squeals?* I admitted my concerns to Mike, and he immediately went out to buy some ex-lax. I read the package, took the suggested dose, waited the appropriate amount of time, and, you guessed it … STILL nothing. *Boy,* I thought uneasily, *this is going to be a MAJOR blow-out when it finally happens.*

I learned a little more since that fateful day, the day I gave birth to a seven-pound clay baby. (Well, okay, I apologize, I don't mean to mislead you. I didn't actually *weigh* the thing, it's just, how else can you fully understand the depths of the pain and effort it took to pass it if you don't visualize a seven-pound clay baby?)

Firstly, I didn't know that you can have two separate issues in this whole constipation department; I thought constipation was only about the bowel being impacted with content that was too hard. I didn't know that you can also experience a motility issue, or sluggish bowels, whereby they are slow to contract and don't actually move. If you have "slow transit constipation" (the lack of high amplitude propagating contractions) or "lazy bowel syndrome," then you also may need a motility drug. I researched a little more and sent Mike back to the store. The post-op literature explained that "sludge" would occur and that it was very important by day five post-op to make sure one had moved their bowels. I sighed. This *was* day five.

I thought and thought about what to do. I couldn't exactly go for a brisk power walk to get things moving, as I was still only at the very beginning of the two-month healing time. Tired of worrying and wondering, I decided I would just sit on the toilet with my feet up, committing to stay there until I had success. And so there I sat. I played on my phone, I read several magazines, and I did a Sudoku puzzle, a hard one (and that takes a while). Worrisomely, still nothing. I sat there a while longer and then unhappily changed my mind. *At this rate I'll be sitting here till the sun comes up.* Reluctantly, I gave up.

And then, to my surprise and joy, the morning of day six I felt an actual *urge* to go. *Finally!* I thought. *Worry over.* Now, without getting into too many details, I will share that during childbirth many years earlier, my body was miserably torn from front to back. To make matters worse, in the post-delivery procedures, the combination of a dimly lit room and an over-enthusiastic intern left me sewn up far too tightly in the posterior. Pair that with occasional constipation and you can well imagine how unpleasant things get at times. *Great*, I thought nervously as I hurried to the toilet, *what the hell is this going to do to my butt?*

And so, sitting on the toilet once more, I proceeded to go into what I can only best describe as "active labour," described as such because there was indeed some panting and blowing, heavy sweating, a bit of screaming and, indescribably severe agony. There was not, however, anyone by my side to squeeze my hand and encourage me, nor was there a cheery nurse mopping my brow, feeding me ice chips and giving me pain meds. I truly wished there had been.

The pain quickly became so severe that it brought me back to my pre-natal training. I started to do my Lamaze breathing, cheeks blowing in and out; —"Hee-hee-hee-hee, whoo-whoo-whoo-whoo"—and I slowly rocked back and forth. I'm not sure if my body naturally responded this way while trying to cope with the pain or if it was me consciously thinking it would get things moving. Either way, it helped a wee bit as I could feel a giant, hard pile sluggishly pushing its way along my much tinier plumbing.

Another minute passed and my toes clenched into tiny bricks of pain and my face twisted as if I were sucking on a lemon. The pain became so severe that I felt like I was borderline passing out. As the hard pile contin-ued to slowly push its way along and the pain got even more intense, I felt like my plumbing had developed, as only a mechanic might best describe, a "cracked cylinder." Now, some of you have experienced childbirth, and some of you have been a partner or a friend supporting someone in that endeavour, and so, for all intents and purposes, I will humiliatingly tell you that this giant poop was now, ahem, "crowning." Unbearably, however, it continued to remain in a "crowned state" with no further momentum and, insufferably, stretching me. It was unequivocally, stuck.

Up to this point, even with having delivered two babies (and having missed the epidural with one of them), this moment was undoubtedly the most painful thing I've ever experienced in all my life. My skin was stretched well beyond its natural diameter and was about to tear. "Mike!" I shouted.

He came running. He looked at me now in concern, my face pale and covered in sweat, my hair stuck to my forehead and cheeks, and the closest he will likely ever get to a woman in "active labor." "Bring me a giant glass of warm water!" I cried out, in between grunts and gasps. He ran off to the kitchen and was back in two seconds flat. I chugged a beer glass full of hot water. I thought the giant amount of water (roughly twenty ounces) would force the poop through the final lag or at least soften it, but I was still not able to completely deliver this horrible clay baby from hell. I was left carefully rocking back and forth as best I could, not able to move much with the sutures, in an attempt to try to push it out or to smoosh it down into a more manageable piece of poop.

That's when I realized it was a solid, rock-hard ball of clay and impossible to get out in the usual manner. Have you ever experienced this? It's terrifying. I had no way to help myself. I tried everything—and I do mean EVERYTHING—to get it out. I was in such agony. It remained there, stubbornly crowning, and my skin slowly started to split. I grabbed onto the corner of the counter as searing hot zaps of nerve pain started coming in waves. I had to do something, and fast. *How could I get this thing out?*

I needed some external help, like a stuck baby needs forceps. I wracked my brain. And then it came to me. (You need to take a deep breath as you read the next part of this terrible story. Once you learn of these next steps, you'll truly understand as I humiliatingly share the oh so suitable quote, "Desperate times call for desperate measures.")

Completely horrified at my own demise, I called Mike back. In a low, slow, husky voice between firmly clenched teeth, I told him to get the Saran Wrap. A brief moment passed between us that I can't really describe. Looking up at him I saw confusion, then realization, and then nausea likely, all crossing his face. He looked down at me pathetically squirming on the porcelain throne and saw desperation, horror, severe pain, and embarrassment. Seventeen years together grants couples the ability to communicate without words, and we both instantly knew how the other was feeling; we both understood what was next.

Off he quickly went, again, back in about two seconds. He handed me the Saran Wrap. "So, is this a *you* thing or a *we* thing?" he asked, even more worried-like. God love him, what an outstanding partner. He was willing to ask, although hesitantly, if I needed him to help.

"It's a *me* thing," I said loudly through deep breaths and still-clenched teeth. Another wave of searing, intense pain swept through me. "Get out!" I yelled. He left. "Well, close the door!" I yelled again in exasperation. *Was this really happening?*

He hurriedly ran back "Sorry, Bubsie," he said, and quickly closed it.

I took a deep breath and pulled the Saran Wrap off the roll, wrapped it around my finger and contemplated how I was actually going to do this. I got the toilet paper ready. "Just like changing a diaper," I coached myself. "I've seen poop before." And less convincingly, "I got this." And, slowly, carefully, unbelievably, I inserted my wrapped finger into my butt. I whimpered in pain as I pushed on the mass and was shocked to discover just how truly solid the poop was. It was harder than my initial thought of extremely firm clay. It was better described as almost concrete. There was no way it was coming out. I pressed on it again. It was legitimately stuck. The Saran Wrap idea wasn't going to work. I tried one last time to move it. Nothing. "Oh my dear God," I cried out, whimpering and desperate, sobbing loudly in agony and panic as complete fear took over, yet still trying hard not to be heard.

My spirits were crushed. How was it that I was actually dealing with even more trauma after the past several days? It was all just too much. I was at the end of my coping skills well before this situation and just needed to recuperate from the surgery itself without trying to hold on, get through, or tough out One. More. Incident.

Screaming now, and unable to reason anymore, I started rolling in circles and rocking back and forth violently, not caring at all about the pressure this caused on all of my internal and external sutures. Squatting and bouncing up and down and grabbing my butt in sheer panic, I desperately tried to get the concrete ball out. I was in tremendous, intense pain. My skin continued to slowly tear, and I became completely desperate to get this awful thing out of me, still very much mimicking active labor.

I looked at the countertop and saw a spoon. It was leftover from the

RestoraLAX I had stirred up in the glass the night before. I thought for a moment. There was no way a spoon would fit in my rectum, but the handle end might. I could insert it a few inches and perhaps maybe move things around, squish it into a smaller mass. I pulled the Saran Wrap off of my finger and, panting heavily to keep from passing out, I grabbed the spoon. In sheer desperation I carefully inserted the end of it to try to scoop out the impacted poo. This was the most painful, horrifying, humiliating, disgusting thing I have ever had to do in my *entire* life. And the spoon handle was not rounded on the handle end. It was square. SQUARE! And it had points on either side. I swear I will never, ever, *for the rest of my life*, look at cutlery the same way.

I tried with all my might to push that stupid clay baby out, and through clenched teeth I screamed and grunted for another five minutes as the damn thing was still only one-quarter of the way out. I was bleeding heavily now, and yet I was no further along. I then got the idea to go to the downstairs toilet where the TUSHY was set up.

Prior to the hysterectomy, Mike had thoughtfully purchased a TUSHY bidet that shoots water up at your bottom when you're on the toilet. The idea is that it saves on toilet paper, keeps you extra clean and fresh, and assists in any painful experiences post-surgery. (It doesn't list that last application but one certainly could use it for that.)

I got up, dizzy now from the exertion. *I'll be lucky if I don't pop a vein in my head,* I nervously thought, breathless from the extended, painful trauma, as well as from the severe anxiety this was causing. I quickly looked at my behind in the mirror and saw that I had a bright pink toilet seat imprinted on the back of my legs and around my butt cheeks. I checked my eyes, fully expecting them to be completely bloodshot from the painful pushing and brutal exertion. I imagined walking Duey and running into the neighbors. "Andrea? What happened to your eyes?" And I would smile and say, "Oh you know, I just birthed a seven-pound clay baby the other day." They'd look at me and awkwardly say "Ohhhhhh." And then I would finish with, "I was in labour for six whole days!"

Down the stairs I went, half praying the clay baby would just decide to drop itself right out on the stairs. *Ah! Wouldn't that be nice?* I hurriedly crossed over the lower room doing the poop walk (up on my tippy-toes, legs spread wide like I just rode a horse for ten days, hand wrapped around behind, just in case.) Even better is that Mike was now on a phone call and watched me as I hobbled by in my dramatic poop walk, naked from the waist down. His mouth dropped open and his eyebrows squelched like he was trying to figure out what was happening, all the while continuing to work, only half-listening now to the guy on the other end of the work call.

I get to the TUSHY and heavily sit down, causing more pain in my abdomen from stitches pulling. I turn it on and am met with icy cold water. We didn't get the deluxe version that had warm water. I mean, why would we? It didn't say on the box, "Purchase the warm water version to assist in the delivery of your seven-pound clay baby."

As I squirm, cold water starts spraying everywhere. I can feel it on my butt cheeks, shooting up my back, and I see water droplets on the wall. I imagine in horror little micro-poop droplets going everywhere, and I quickly turn TUSHY off. At this point, I would guess that this whole experience from beginning to end spanned about an hour, so I decided to turn TUSHY back on—messy or not, and cold anyway—as I just couldn't take another second of this hell. Suddenly I felt the powerful cold water jet stream go up inside me, *through* the poo. *Likely through the hole I made with the spoon*, I realize, and I shuddered as I tried to erase the thought.

The cold water made my insides contract, and I felt my bowels stinging with the onset of more micro tears as my outer skin again stretched well beyond its natural design, completely destroying my butt. "Dear GOD Get this thing out of me!" I heard myself yell. My body took over and, with one giant heave and a single, jungle-like animal grunt that could have competed with a woman pushing out a *thirteen*-pound baby, the heavens opened up and I finally pooped out that glorious hard-pack son-of-a-gun. SPLASH!

"Finally!" I yelled. "I birthed the clay baby! It's out! Whoo hoo!" I cheered and smiled in celebration and was able to ignore the residual pain as I was so overjoyed and immensely relieved in that very epic moment. In classic, true Andrea form, in my mind I heard the celebratory music that only rings out in triumphant moments such as this—a full compilation of big brassy trumpets and a choir of angels loudly singing, "Haaaallelujah! Hallelujah! Hallelujah!"

And so I sat there, panting and recovering for several minutes. Now having finally birthed it I almost expected Mike to come around the corner carrying helium balloons and to wrap the clay baby in a birthing blanket. He'd pass it to me along with a big, fat, Cuban cigar while shaking my hand in congratulations.

And with that horrific moment now over, I thought perhaps all of the trauma from the past several months would come to an end. I wondered now, would life *finally* return to normal? I was hopeful. But nope, not even remotely close. You see, my friends, this was the beginning of a fresh new hell, the very large, very angry, external hemorrhoid that would miserably plague me for the next six months. I should've told Mike to buy stock in Preparation H. When all was said and done, I think I must've gone through a thousand boxes, maybe more.

You likely now understand why we are warned about the dangers of severe constipation. I hope no one ever again has to experience what I went through. My situation was extreme, dangerous, and hugely painful. Both the internal and external damage was and still is, extensive.

Following the clay-baby delivery, the perfectly normal thing to do next would be to have a hot shower, take some Tylenol, poor a stiff drink, and head to bed. But me? What did I do? I called my sister. She answered and I skipped all formalities and started in with, "Lara. You are *not* going to believe THIS!"

20

THE SAGA CONTINUES

In great detail I described the past hour. Lara was in complete hysterics, laughing uncontrollably and repeatedly yelling, "No way! No waaaaay!" as I rambled on. Telling her my disgusting, shocking, unthinkable experience and hearing her whooping and laughing in hysterics was not only enough to get me roaring in giant, guttural outbursts, but also enough to cause me to bend over (painfully) in half, tears rolling down my face and head bobbing silently up and down. Lara's laugh is infectious and I am filled with joy whenever she and I giggle together. I felt proud that I had survived yet another horror.

Once we settled, she told me she was still bleeding and was wondering if she was having the equivalent of "sympathy pains." I recalled her telling me while I was in hospital the week before that she hadn't had a period in two years and yet all of a sudden she was bleeding heavily. Like, "birthing a bat" kinda heavily. My adrenalin started pumping hard and I felt very scared for her. We hung up and I researched things for a few minutes. I called her back in a hurry. "Lara," I said, "from the symptoms you've shared, this sounds like it could be ovarian cancer. Call your doc a.s.a.p." Mere hours later, I witnessed the true miracle of the US medical system. Not only was she at her doctor's the very next day, but inside of a week she was scheduled for a complete hysterectomy dated for two weeks from the doctor's appointment, March first. What took me almost *two years* total from first symptoms to my organs out, would mind-blowingly only take my sister three and a half weeks. Incredibly, the timing meant my poor mother now had to deal with both of her daughters having major surgeries within a month of one another, and a second daughter dealing with a cancer threat. At times, it's crazy how life plays out.

Valentine's Day came and went, and I wondered when Dr. Scott was going to call me with the results of my own hysterectomy. I was starting to wonder if perhaps everything was normal and therefore I would not receive a phone call. The next day, Mike went out for a grocery order and my phone rang.

"Andrea?" a voice said.

Hesitantly I responded, "Yes?"

"This is Dr. Scott calling. How are you doing?"

I was relieved it was her but also didn't recognize her voice; it was not her usual warm and relaxed tone that I had become so accustomed to. I briefly told her about the labour-and-delivery episode (but out of respect to her I chose not to refer to it as the seven-pound clay baby) and mentioned a few other things like the fact that my stitches were still very red, itchy, crusty, and not dissolving. She told me to come in to see her and she would remove them, and I thought we were going to say goodbye.

But then she dropped a completely unexpected bomb. "Andrea, do you remember when I saw you in recovery after your hysterectomy and I mentioned that there was a grey, shady spot on one of your ovaries in the scan and that we couldn't make out what it was?"

Instantly, my blood stopped. I swallowed hard. "Yes." I couldn't breathe.

"Is anybody with you right now?" she asked.

"No, Mike is out getting groceries." *Shit-shit-shit-shit-shit-shit-shit.*

"Okay, well we did the biopsies and dissected the ovary and it looks like the cancer has spread."

This, my good people, was undoubtedly the most terrifying news I have ever received in all of my fifty-one years. Genuinely. My mind started racing. My pulse was so fast I thought my heart was going to rattle into oblivion, and I knew my blood pressure was sky-rocketing.

"The good news is that we didn't find any cancer in the lymph nodes we took out, and we took out sixteen or so, but it *did* spread to your left ovary." *No it did not.* "So you have definitely had this cancer for a very long time, as it is a slow-growing type of cancer. We're now upgrading you to stage and grade 3a." *Oh my God. Isn't stage four terminal? And I'm now at stage three?* "This means you will need to do chemo and radiation." My mind went completely numb at this point, and I started slowly hyperventilating. "Can you come in and we will meet with the team and go over everything?"

Slight pause. "Yes," I said quietly, now going into shock again, not unlike that fateful day last November. But this news was so much worse. *Chemo? Radiation? This was too surreal. Please God, wake me up from this nightmare.* "When?" I asked. *This is NOT happening. This isn't real.*

"I'd like you to come in this Friday. The booking office will call you. Do you have any questions?" She sounded more relaxed when she said this.

I can't imagine being in a job where you have to tell people such horrible news on a regular basis. "Uh, when will I likely start all of the treatments?" I asked, dreading the answer, now stammering and completely terrified.

"Probably in April. You will be mostly healed then from your hysterectomy."

"Okay, uh, I was to start a new job as a spa concierge. Is this something I can still do?" I had no clue. No. Clue.

"No, you will not feel well enough to work. I am so sorry." We hung up after another few minutes.

I lay on my couch, completely dumbfounded—literally. I could not speak or produce a thought. And I was going to have to resign from my dream job. A brand new spa was opening and I had completed training back in December and couldn't wait to start as the spa concierge. It was a three-minute drive from our home on the ocean. Now I was forced to quit the dream job that never was. I lay there, trying to make sense of it all. At times like these, one wonders what one has done to end up with the universe dealing such a raw, hateful hand. I once knew a marathon runner who was the epitome of health, and to the devastation of the whole community, she died at thirty-six from an aggressive cancer. I lay there in mind-numbing sadness as the questions started coming, fast and furious: *Why is this happening to me? I am a good person. I treat people decently. I am honest and kind. Why is my life falling apart?*

Just then Mike came in with armloads of grocery bags, took one look at me, and dropped them all on the floor.

"What's going on now?" he asked, crossing the room in about two strides.

"Dr. Scott called." Hearing my voice tremble, I paused for a second, trying to get my emotions in check. I didn't want to upset Mike any more than was necessary. "My cancer spread to one of my ovaries, so now they have to do chemo and radiation. I'm upgraded to 3a." *An "upgrade." Why is this called an upgrade? Usually we love upgrades—a better hotel room, a first-class seat on the plane, a nicer table at a fine restaurant. I want to go back to the level 1 stage. THAT would be an upgrade.*

Mike scratched his head and expelled a large amount of air. "But, your ovaries came out with the hysterectomy, didn't they? Why chemo and radiation?"

This is the question I would come to explain to a million people a thousand-billion times in the next several months.

"It's preventative. It's just in case a rogue cancer cell broke through and is metastasizing somewhere else."

"Okay. So, you don't *know* if it is anywhere else, it's just preventative. Okay. Okay. So, what are you thinking?" He looked at me, his face pretty stoic. "It's preventative, so are you feeling like you want to go through with this?" He asked me so gently and carefully; he was truly the most thoughtful of partners.

I tried to think. "I don't really know *what* to make of this. I mean, I don't want to *not* do it and then find it has spread to my liver, my lungs, my brain . . . but chemo and radiation are so hard on the body. It's awful!" My shock started to subside and the tears started to flow. Heavily. I just could not understand that this nightmare was mine. "She wants us to come in on Friday to talk about it all."

And, again, we just sort of went quietly about our business, trying to absorb another blow. Mike put the groceries away and I went back to watching movies in the guest room. I was only fifteen days into healing from the hysterectomy, and I still felt very sore and mentally exhausted.

Friday came and we met with Dr. Scott. She took her time explaining the process, and I felt confident that I could fully trust her opinion and knowledge. I was quite terrified to even be contemplating the chemo and radiation. The thought of poisons in my body and all the awful stories we've all heard over the years just sounded so completely terrible. But, there was no way around it. Even though it was preventative, it was too risky to chance there being a rogue cell or two waiting elsewhere in my body to start up again. Dr. Scott explained that I would be getting the "chemo sandwich," whereby I would do four doses of chemo, then switch to twenty-five radiation treatments and two brachytherapy treatments, followed by more chemo after that. "Likely two more, to be clear."

At this point in my cancer journey, I simply thought that chemo was chemo, like Tylenol is Tylenol—one type and just a few strengths. Now I know that there are well over one hundred types of chemo, various combinations of them used together, and various dosages based on your body weight and stage of cancer. I was to receive Carboplatin and Paclitaxel. At first I couldn't remember the names at all, but after a bit I became quite well versed in them, spelling them off like I was queen of the spelling bees. Brachytherapy scared me the most, as it is internal radiation in the vagina. I just could not get my head around any of this.

"So, is the chemo oral?" I asked, hopeful.

"No, the chemo is every three weeks, and you will come here to the Dickson Centre to get an IV.

Oh no. I'm terrible with IVs! "Okay. Why is it every three weeks?" I asked, having no clue how this would impact me.

"The chemo needs time to do its thing and for you to recover from it. Each round of chemo, we check that your neutrophils are okay and that all of your blood work looks good. It takes about three weeks to come up each time from the infusion." I hastily jotted down notes on the pad of paper I had brought. "You will also need to monitor your temperature. If you get any fever at all, you need to come right in and get checked out."

Oh wow. "Okay, if that happens, do I call you? Or what do I do?" I truly had no idea.

"You will go to emerg."

"And wait for eight hours?"

"No. Cancer patients get this yellow card. It has all of the instructions and medications you would need to take, typed on the back, in case you develop any kind of infection. Protocol dictates that you will be seen within thirty minutes of arriving at emerg. You cannot risk waiting as it can escalate pretty quickly and potentially become life-threatening if you get a bacterial infection. Low neutrophils mean you cannot fight off infection on your own and you can go downhill very fast." I gasped audibly as she continued. "Check your temp each morning and if it is up at all, check it again in thirty minutes, and come in right away if it is elevated higher than 100.4 Fahrenheit." I looked over the laminated, yellow card and placed it in my bag.

Okay, I thought. *I almost never get fevers, so chances are unlikely that I will get one.*

"Here is your blood requisition. You need to keep this somewhere safe as you will use the same paper for the next six months. You will need to get blood work every three weeks. You are to book it as close as you can to the day of your chemo treatment. So if you are booked on a Tuesday, get it on the Sunday or the Monday."

I was overwhelmed by the amount of information thrown at me, most of which I had never heard before. She put her hand on my arm.

"Andrea, I know this is a lot. You are going to be okay. The chemo works. It is the best route to go, and the staff at the Cancer Centre are excellent."

Dr. Scott was truly the best doctor I have ever dealt with. I teared up, feeling overwhelmed by how blessed I was to be in her care. I told her this and she humbly accepted my words as we finished up.

We were told that Nurse Jess would call in the next few days once I had read over the information booklets. I had about twelve different ones to read. It was a lot to take in, and I was scared and still very much in denial about the whole process.

On the long drive home my mind returned to the conversation in Dr.

Scott's office. "Will I lose my hair?" I had asked, and was so scared to hear the answer. My hair was my prized possession. I had worn it long for years, and it was an auburn red that I thought was fun and unique. It gave me security and also self-confidence.

"Yes. With these drugs, you will lose your hair. Likely within the first few weeks." Her eyes looked sad, like she too could understand my grief. She herself had beautiful, long, thick hair.

"Oh wow," I said, utterly disappointed. *This is horrible. Maybe it's only a little hair loss.* "How much hair will I lose?" I asked, so SO hopeful that maybe it was only a wee bit.

"All of it," she said, looking even sadder for me now. She must really hate these appointments. *I'm going to be bald? Noooo.*

"So, like, *completely* bald?"

"Yes."

"Like an egg?"

"Like an egg."

I felt like I had been punched in the stomach. *How will I deal with this? Now I definitely will look like I have cancer.*

"So, how does the radiation work?" I was almost ready to run out the door at this point.

"You will have radiation for a few minutes every day, Monday to Friday, for about five weeks. You will have a different oncologist for that. They will contact you and go over the details and make sure everything is lined up. That will be in a few months from now; we do the four chemo sessions first." She wrote the numbers down in front of me. "Chemo is three-week intervals, four rounds, so that's about twelve weeks. So, yes, likely about June you will start radiation."

I was stunned. I factored in the time in between, plus the last two chemo rounds. I was going to lose my whole summer, wouldn't be golfing with my friends, swimming, sailing, or doing any of the stuff I thoroughly loved to do. I had been dreaming of kayaking and paddling around with Duey from our new home. This barrage of treatment torture was going to be my life for at least the next seven months. It sounded exhausting.

We thanked Dr. Scott for her thoroughness and her patience and left the Cancer Centre feeling apprehensive and afraid and with far too much to think about.

We drove most of the way to our home in silence yet again, both deep in thought. I called my family pretty much right away, but of course, I severely down played the news. I did not share the "upgrade" to stage 3a with any of them; it sounded way too scary.

A few days later I turned to my social media friends for more support.

Social Media Post #3
February 26

♡ *update* ♡

Well folks, looks like the cancer train isn't done with me yet. The surgeon didn't like the pathology results, and now I've got seven months of chemo and radiation coming up. I've been trying hard to keep up with all the check-ins, phone calls, messages, and visits but am finding I can't be on my phone that much and just want to sleep, so please know I love you and I am so, so touched and grateful for your messages; I just can't reply to them all as thoroughly as I'd like. Anyhow. I'm not dying, to be clear. This is as a prevention so that we can make sure no more little cancer cells settle and cause trouble. So. If you've done chemo, shoot me a private message of any tips or success stories please, and know that, as many of you have already said, "I got this!!"

♡ ♡ ♡

Again, the outpouring of messages was incredible. I was filled with hope and an overwhelming sense of love from all of the communication. I was also very surprised to learn that at least five of my friends had also gone through cancer. I did not know this. Some of them had had chemo, some had radiation, some had surgery and opted not to have chemo, but all of them offered words of support and wisdom, and I treasured it all. Some people told me I was brave, sharing my journey on social media. I was surprised. Why wouldn't I share? My friends and family were all so very worried and asking a barrage of questions each and every day, and I thought it was a great way to efficiently reach everyone. It never crossed my mind that some people would choose to handle this privately. I certainly couldn't, not with the very large circle I kept up with. I didn't want to continually have to explain why my hair was gone every time I ran into someone, and I certainly didn't want to have to avoid people. Besides, social media should not always be about living the fabricated, "perfectly happy" life. We need to share the "downs," not just the perfectly happy "ups."

21
BOXING GLOVES

Lara and I continued to FaceTime each other every day. She was always checking in, and I was keeping her informed of the delicacies and intricacies of the healing, as her surgery was coming up fast and would be a similar procedure. She said she was grateful for all that I shared.

One night, the simple action of just getting up from the couch seemed too much, and I realized Lara would appreciate a video of humour, to help her manage through some of the more painful logistics she would soon have. I grabbed my phone, pushed the "record" button, and handed it to Mike. With a silly wig, a British accent and speaking like a senior, I described step by step how one must execute such an awkward, painful task of getting up off the couch from a lying down position when full of sutures. I added grunts, profanities, and fart noises to keep it humorous even though it was a painful, frustrating struggle.

"Welcome to the how-to-get-the-f*ck-off-the-couch-after-the-hysterectomy video," I started. My accent was similar to Maggie Smith's in *Downton Abbey*, and I expertly rolled my *R*'s.

"Step one: Fart now, so you don't embarrass yourself later." (I lifted my leg and blew an obnoxious, loud, fake fart, feigning embarrassment afterward.)

"Step two: Carefully roll to the side." (I grunt, curse, roll, and moan with over exaggerated effort while delivering a perfectly executed roll of the *R* once again.)

"Step 3: If you are on your r-r-r-r-right side, use your left hand to push yourself up into a sitting position on the couch," (more loud groans, fart noises, and swear words) "and carefully come to an upright position." It was indeed a struggle, by now my wig was sideways, and I left it like that for more laughs.

"Step 4: Sit like a big, fat sumo wrestler." (I opened my thighs as wide as they would allow and placed my hands on my legs, my elbows bent outward. I grunt, wig now covering half my face, and I fart some more.)

"Step 5: Carefully shimmy your buttocks to the edge of the couch." (I shimmy, awkwardly, carefully, noisily as I continue to swear and grunt.)

"Step 6: Use the non-existent muscles in your thighs to then flex up off of the couch." (I groan heavily as if I am having a baby and push up with more exaggerated effort in the best yogi-sumo standing position I can get into.)

"Step 7: Wave your arms around while saying in your best Elvis impression, 'Thank you, thank you, thank you very much.'"

I finished the act and began giggling. I asked Mike to send the video off to Lara while I continued to giggle. Having wrapped the filming, he shook his head and told me I was a complete nut.

Even though I was able to add humour to my situation, I continued to have a great deal of pain in my abdomen and wondered when I would be able to bend properly to shave my legs, pick up the dog bowls, or even retrieve things I had dropped. Each time I bent, I felt a deep pain in my lower left side.

A few days later, we drove to the hospital again. I had to go back to see Dr. Scott for my four-week post-op checkup, and she did the internal. It was quite painful. "Don't put anything in there for another four weeks," she instructed.

"Trust me, I won't. I'm terrified," I grimly replied. I had done some research about the female anatomy. I looked at diagrams to understand more about how I was impacted by the surgery. The cervix is at the top of the vagina, so when the uterus, ovaries, tubes, and cervix are all removed, the top of the vagina has to be stitched so that it remains closed. I was deeply bothered by that idea and was afraid that any type of penetration would tear the stitches. I was quite happy to wait a bit longer.

Four weeks into my own post-op, my sister went in for her hysterectomy in California. Within two hours of her operation, they had analyzed a suspicious tumour. Her husband, Douglas, called and, much to our relief, said the doctors reported there was no cancer. I was confused by how quickly he had this information. *This can't be right*, I thought. *How could they know already? It took sixteen days for me to get my results.* I asked my own oncology team how it was that Lara was able to know within hours of her surgery. It was an eye-opener for us to learn that it shouldn't ever take two weeks. It is indeed possible to determine the state of tissue health within the same day, but for Nova Scotians, the labs are just that backed up.

While I was Face Timing with Lara the next day, I said, "I'm so happy for you! What a huge relief that you don't have cancer!" Her face started to move in an odd sort of way, and then she started to cry. "Lara, what's wrong?" I asked, scared there was something bad she wasn't telling me.

She struggled a bit to share her feelings. "Oh, Andrea. I'm just so overwhelmed with sadness. It's not right that my doctors were able to deal with my health issues so quickly and that they could remove the tumor and do my hysterectomy right away, and yet you had to wait so ridiculously long to finally get a diagnosis. I feel guilty that I was able to be seen in a timely manner and that I managed to dodge this horrible disease, and yet you have suffered and struggled so much because of such a bogged-down health care system. You could've avoided all of this had they seen you in time." She thought for a moment longer. "You're going through so much more than me. It's just not fair." She took another deep breath and struggled again at sharing her thoughts. I waited for her to continue and tried hard not to cry while I watched her face change with all of the emotion she was feeling.

"I wish you didn't have cancer. I actually feel guilty that I don't have it. If we both had the same diagnosis, you wouldn't have to be going through all of this alone." Her voice started to waver. She put her hand over her mouth and stifled a sob. She was miserable. "I wish I had it too, or that I could take yours for you." I watched her body jerk with more sobs that she desperately tried to contain.

I was completely blown away. Those words embedded themselves right on my heart. I was at a loss for words, and a few moments passed before I gently pleaded, "Lara, don't ever wish that you had cancer. This is *my* path and *my* lesson. For some reason I am deemed to learn something from this and to go through this. I truly believe everything happens for a reason. It'll be okay. *I'll* be okay. I promise." We talked a bit more and then we hung up.

The depth of that conversation and all that she shared solidified my understanding of her commitment to me as my older, guardian sister. I was blinded by her true, demonstrative love and compassion for me; I had never known she felt that strong.

A few days later two cookbooks showed up on my doorstep. They were hardcover and incredibly well written. They were created specifically for cancer patients and had everything from preparing what to eat before chemo began, to what to eat during and after treatments. They even had sections such as "Nausea and Low Appetite," "Low Platelets," and "Energy and Dehydration." These books were wondrous and greatly informative. Lara had sent them. She explained that she had a friend in Boston who had gone through cancer and that these books were very helpful to her friend, and so she purchased them for me. Even from 6,000 kilometres away, Lara still had my back and I felt grateful to receive these gifts.

Five weeks post-op, International Women's Day arrived. Various people were posting about women's rights and achievements. I thought about my upcoming hair loss and the stigma that accompanies bald women. I thought about the pressure to look perfectly put together and how so many people spend a great deal of time using filters to make themselves look flawless. It bothers me a great deal, the pressures we place on ourselves as a society to constantly seek perfection. I decided to let my friends know that I was going to be bald.

Social Media Post #4

March 8

> Happy International Women's Day! In just a few short weeks I will be completely bald, due to chemo. It's been a rough week accepting that. But, pardon the pun, I think I'm starting to "get my head around it." Inner strength is a gift. And I want to show others that

> it's ok to put your vulnerable side out there. When I'm able, I'll post
> a real baldy pic. ♡

The chemo-countdown was on as I slowly continued to recover from my hysterectomy. I was still plagued with severe night sweats as my hormones had indeed taken a nosedive with the ovaries suddenly gone. I was also still in a great amount of pain and continued to experience tremendous fatigue. I napped regularly yet I was barely getting enough sleep. I was immensely worried about the upcoming treatments, and physically I just couldn't get comfortable. Being a stomach sleeper was still not permitted, and, as hard as I tried, I could not manage to get into a comfortable position on either my side or my back. My abdomen remained quite swollen, and I was challenged to do anything physical at all. Frustratingly, I still could not bend over, could not tie my own shoes or even manage to put on my own socks. I had to wear big billowy dresses; as any type of waistband hurt me very badly. (The downside of being a fair-skinned redhead made for a delicate, scarring mess both inside and out.)

Not being able to drive for a full eight weeks' post-op meant I was pretty much housebound. In fact, I had been housebound since January first, as the COVID-19 pandemic was still alive and well, so I had chosen to isolate. I didn't want any potential chance of COVID causing an issue for my surgical date. So, with those four weeks in January waiting at home for surgery, and then the additional eight weeks of healing, I was starting to feel quite challenged mentally. I spent a great amount of time in the little guest room just lying in bed, pondering life. I watched a great deal of TV, trying to keep my mind off both my current situation and the upcoming one. Fighting off misery, I was running dangerously low on coping skills. I worked tremendously hard at staying positive, as it would have been very easy to slip into a severe depression—and *that* scared me more than anything.

Thankfully, over the next few weeks I had many friends and family dropping by to see me. Each time, people would bring me coffee, tea, or little gifts. It was truly heart-warming, and I was grateful for all of the blessings people bestowed upon us.

A few more days went by and then another delivery came to our house. Mike took the box and then was immediately on the phone, speaking quietly to someone. He came over and said, "Your sister wants to FaceTime you." I had been crying and didn't feel like talking. I had low energy, was stressed about the chemo starting, and was just plain down in the dumps. I tried to avoid the FaceTime, and Mike said, "Just talk to her, it'll cheer you up."

I got on the phone. Lara was all smiles and said, "I sent something for you!"

Mike brought over the boxed package. *Another* gift? "Is it another cookbook?" I asked.

"Nope." She kept smiling. "Just open it."

I opened the package. It was a light-pink cashmere poncho.

"That's for you!" Lara said, just so excited. "Each time you wear it, know that I'm there with you giving you a great big hug! Maybe even wear it on chemo day."

I was in tears at this point. Douglas came into view as Mike brought yet another box over.

"I know I sent you cookbooks and the poncho but I wanted to get you one more thing. Here's your last gift!" Lara said. She was really excited.

Mike began playing "This is my Fight Song" by Rachel Platten as I opened the package. To my amazement, I was looking at bubble-gum pink, ladies boxing gloves. *Actual boxing gloves!* I was completely blown away. I started ugly crying, realizing the thoughtful symbolism of this gift; it represented so much.

"Andrea, we know you have the fight of your life coming up. And with your spirit and your positivity, we know you've got this. These gloves are to remind you to fight hard and to be strong and to never give up and to know how much we love you." Lara was beaming pure love.

Well. Ugly cry ensued, now paired with giant heaving body spasms, loud wails, and a full-on snot-fest. My grief overtook me and I started wailing even louder. Deep, guttural, animal cries and body spasms and giant tears and snot all over my face. I was a complete mess. And I was embarrassed. No one sees me like this. Ever. Well, except maybe Mike on a rare occasion.

I tried hard to pull myself together but just couldn't. I put the gloves on. They fit perfectly; like . . . a glove. "I'm going to wear these on my first day." I said through huffs and puffs and sniffles. I had bought a pair of pink camouflage leggings and thought these would go perfectly.

"Excellent!" Lara and Douglas said, the two of them also crying. Douglas added, "Andrea, I love you, and from what I can see, you are in the right frame of mind. You are doing really well and handling things just so positively. You got this." I saw tears in his eyes; he, too, genuinely cared. It was such an incredible, moving moment between the four of us.

"Lara, I always wanted to box. Do you remember when we were kids and we were in Jennifer's basement and there was a white cloth bag hanging from the beams full of stuff? I thought it was a punching bag for boxing, and I pulled back, wound up and slammed my fist right into the bag as hard as I could, only to learn that it was her brother David's hockey bag. I had slammed my fist right into his helmet!"

She cracked up laughing, "Uh, vaguely, yes." She smiled, shaking her head at the memory of me in my youth. I ended up spraining my wrist that day and severely bruising my knuckles. I was excused from piano lessons for two weeks.

I looked back at the gifts. The gloves were fabulous. We hung them up where I could see them each day and could be reminded in my lowest of lows to be strong and to fight. I started to get my head around the fact that I had an enormously tough battle coming up, and coming up fast.

PART TWO

22

BYE-BYE, LOCKS

Chemo was scheduled to begin in late March, the day after Maddie's birthday celebration.

It is interesting to reflect on the emotions I had around losing my hair. I was unaware that it was so very much a part of all of my emotions. I often used it as a tool to hide behind; if I was naked, I kept my long locks in front of me, to give me some privacy as my body inevitably aged. If I felt a little insecure, my hair served as a giant lion's mane. If I felt adventurous, a big, boofy bun on the top of my head showed everyone my playful mood. If I was dressing up, I could look more glamorous with my hair piled high with little wisps pulled down around my face.

Knowing my hair was going to all fall out was terrifying. What if I had an ugly, weird mark on my scalp from all of my wipeouts as a kid? Many a time I had required stitches as I flipped over the handlebars of my bike. Or what if, as it grew in, I looked like a giant strawberry with all of the red bristly bits? Or even worse, what if my dear husband found me repulsive? These concerns kept me up at night.

I decided to join a chemotherapy and radiation support group online. It was a wealth of information, some good and some bad. The more I researched, the more I learned that my hair was likely going to fall out between day ten and day fourteen after the first round. *Wow that's coming up fast . . .* I thought, with great sadness. I also read that it was better to cut it down short so that it would be less upsetting; people with long hair said it was quite unnerving to have giant long clumps of hair falling out all over the bedsheets, the pillow, while in the shower, taking a bath, on the front of your sweater and in your hands. I knew I did not want to cut my hair off—I thought I might look like a boy—but the alternative was certainly not optimal!

People asked me if I was going to shave my head. *Gosh!* That sounded *way* too ambitious, and as I researched further, I learned that if you shave it down clean with a blade, the little hair follicles get trapped in your scalp and then become inflamed, infected, painful, red, and rashy. All of this, so unpleasant.

So, in typical Andrea style, I faced my new reality head-on and made a plan to hold a "hair-chopping ceremony."

Because we live so far out of the city, it did not make sense to have my family drive out once for Maddie's birthday, and then again a few days later for the hair ceremony, and I knew after chemo started that I would likely not even feel up to it then, so I planned both for the same day. We celebrated Maddie's birthday first, as I wanted to have my hair looking normal for her birthday pics.

No one knew of my hair plans yet. I must admit, I felt a little distracted and uncertain about my secret plans during her birthday, but again, I did my best to keep my emotions in check and smiled my way through presents and cake. I didn't want to upset my girls on such a special day.

After the birthday had been fully celebrated and our bellies were full of cake, I walked over to the kitchen and promptly got four pairs of scissors and some hair elastics. My family looked at me curiously. I tried so darn hard not to get emotional as I explained what the situation was with my hair. Suddenly things got real, very fast. My girls and my mother looked at me with such mixed emotions. They undoubtedly felt sad and concerned as the worry over my upcoming chemo started to hit them, but I knew they also felt proud. Proud to see how strong I was; proud to see me being brave, even though they knew how troubling it was for me to lose my hair. They tried to hide their emotions, and their faces quivered with effort. The guys looked awkward and squirmed a bit, as they too tried to hide their great discomfort and heavy emotion.

"So!" I said, all teacher-like. "Here's the plan! I'm going to divide my hair into four ponytails and a mohawk section on top, and then Mom, Annie, Maddie, you three are going to each take scissors and cut off the ponytails with me!" They looked at me like I was nuts. I think they wondered what the scene would be once the hair was off. Was I going to cry? Would I hate how I looked? They certainly didn't have any time to prepare themselves for this unexpected moment so were also struggling to deal with this big, upsetting surprise. They were gracious. "Then, we are going to get the guys to use the clippers and neaten things up over the ears and back of the neck. Oh! I almost forgot! We are going to record this so that I can share this with others in the cancer community who may benefit from seeing it."

I smiled and looked around, half-excited. I'd always wanted a mohawk. When I was in high school back in the late '80s, we had various groups—the nerds, the head bangers, the band kids, the punks, the populars—and there was this one punk girl, Darlene, who'd had a mohawk that was dyed black and about eighteen inches long. It was incredible. She put egg white and gel in it every day and would show up with it either all standing up in one shiny, beautiful, bird-like feather design, or she'd divide it into six spiked segments and wear those pointy bits straight up. It was truly fascinating and a work of art.

One day the school decided Darlene was no longer allowed to wear her mohawk, claiming the spikes were "dangerous, sharp, and weapon-like," and the straight mohawk was "too distracting for other students." I felt so sad when she had to stop wearing it, and I always said that in an alternate world, I would plan on having one. So, lo and behold, today was the day.

I put on my bright pink, tie-dyed dress, grabbed my pink boxing gloves from Lara and Douglas for props, and began to section my hair off in quadrants. I had Alicia Keys' song "This Girl is on Fire!" playing in the background to give me courage.

The room was pretty quiet considering there were seven of us there plus Duey. People were feeling really emotional at this point as the reality of the long journey ahead and the current state of my health was really starting to sink in. In essence, we were about to say goodbye to the girl with the long red hair we'd all known for what seemed like forever.

"Are you sure this is what you want to do?" Mom asked, looking a little nervous for me.

"Well, I don't really have a choice, Ma, so, yup. We're doing it!" Once again, I played the role of cheerleader and Miss Positive, trying to make the best of it.

They each took a ponytail and held it in their hands. The music played and the guys held their phones up, waiting to record. "Okay!" I yelled, "We're gonna do this on the count of three!"

"Wait!" someone said. "Is three when we begin to cut or is three when we are to be done and holding up the ponytails?"

"I don't know!" I yelled. "Just cut!" My adrenalin was pumping. "Guys. Begin filming!" Phones went on. "Okay, so, hi, everyone, my name's Andrea, I live in Nova Scotia, and I have endometrial cancer. I start chemo tomorrow and I am about to cut off all of my hair. I have had long hair my entire life, and I am cutting it off to begin my cancer journey. I want everyone to know that it is no big deal, it's okay, it's just hair!" I couldn't think of anything else to say; I was nervous and trying not to cry. "Okay! Here we go. One, two, three!" I reached up and found my ponytail and began cutting. I could feel the others' scissors cutting away. My head bobbed from side to side as the hands holding my ponytails pulled and moved with strength trying to time it right to get the hair off simultaneously.

Of course, my scissors were dull. "Ok! I got it!" someone exclaimed, and held up a ponytail. Another one seconds later, "Me too!" And then another. With the long hair gone, my head felt really light. I continued to hack away with my dull scissors, and then Annie offered to cut with me. Finally, we got the last one off. I held it up in the air triumphantly, like the scene of the newborn cub in the musical *The Lion King*. I yelled "Whoo hoo! We did it!" and then I sat there breathless and teary with four ponytails in my lap. Fourteen eyes staring at me, taking in the change. I looked at their faces, trying to discern what they were thinking.

"Is it awful?" I asked; I had no mirror around me.

"No! It actually looks really cute!" the girls said.

"Good God, Andrea, you have a perfectly shaped head. You look beautiful." My mother smiled.

I ran to the bathroom. I was surprised. I actually *did* look pretty cute. I still had the top section of hair that I had saved for the mohawk, and it flopped to one side. I smiled at myself. It wasn't so bad.

"Okay! Out to the porch to shave the back!" I directed. The guys looked a little unsure. "C'mon! We're doing this!" So, out we all went, this time with the girls videoing, while Mike, Dad, and Kyle all took turns using the electric shaver to neaten me up. It was an extraordinary moment, and also sort of a great send-off for the journey I was about to embark upon.

We went inside and hung out, and after a little while longer, it was time for everyone to return to the city. There were lots of hugs and they all wished me luck. They knew that in less than twenty-four hours I would have my first dose of chemo. As the door closed behind them, I quietly turned around, walked quickly to the bathroom, and once more, bawled my eyes out.

23
MOHAWK

Some time later, I took a deep breath, cleaned my face up, and with great effort pulled myself together to re-focus. I went to the kitchen and began trying to design my mohawk. I got out some eggs and began separating them. I dug out the beaters and started whipping the whites. Mike came over. "Whatcha makin'?" he asked, thinking perhaps something yummy. *Mmm. Meringues would be great right about now.*

"Oh just whipping up some egg whites for my hair." I said, a little devilishly.

He scrunched his face. "Egg whites?"

He didn't say more as I gave him a look. I'd done some research on how to best get your hair hard and to stand on end.

"I'm gonna put this in my hair and blow-dry it." I smiled; I couldn't wait. My head being freshly coiffed, I had a soft mohawk of four-inch hair hanging sideways. I planned to divide it into six quadrants and spike them like my high school friend. I was going to walk into the Cancer Centre like a BOSS. I continued beating the egg whites until they formed stiff peaks; I squealed with delight. I ran with the bowl to the bathroom and dunked my hands into the egg whites. I had forgotten that they have a slight smell. I blobbed the egg whites into my hair and started running my hands all the way through the four inches, carefully and methodically working the eggs in. Then I got a comb and sectioned it all off and put ponytail elastics in the sections to divide each one. Next I began blow-drying my hair.

The heat of the hairdryer almost instantly turned my hands super sticky, and I could feel them beginning to stick to it. My hair, on the other hand, didn't get sticky at all but rather turned slimy and hot. I couldn't get the one small piece of each hair segment to stand straight up. I pulled my sticky hands off the hairdryer and washed them. Then I carefully undid the five other elastics and decided to blow-dry it all together while upside down to see if that would do the trick. Within a mere matter of seconds, my hands became hot and itchy, once again sticking to the dryer. My hair suddenly got stuck together and started to turn white and flaky. The egg whites were not performing at all like I had expected. I grabbed my hairbrush and ran it through my hair, trying to get it to wrap around the brush and to then harden. No go. My hair got stuck in the brush and bits of white, dried egg started caking in the bristles.

Mike appeared and leaned against the bathroom door. "Are you sure this is how it's supposed to go?" he asked kindly. I looked at him in frustration. My arms were getting tired.

"No, it was supposed to harden instantly and be perfect by now!"

He looked thoughtful. "Maybe wash that stuff out and try some glue?" So, I stripped down, grabbed a quick shower, dried off and went looking for glue. I recalled just a few days before that I had come across five glue sticks while looking for the special paper to make Maddie's birthday card. I found them and tried one. It was completely dried out. I proceeded to try each and every one of them only to discover they were *all* dried out. "Oh for Pete's sake!" I sighed, pitching them at the garbage can. On to Plan C. Liquid glue. I dug it out and globbed it in. I carefully started to blow-dry it. It congealed into one giant, stuck pile of hair not unlike a rat's nest. I tried patiently to pull it all apart again and I carefully teased it with a comb. I was getting cold; the house was drafty in late March. I was standing there in my bathrobe as I hadn't taken the time to properly dress after I had showered— I was too excited. My arms were starting to quiver a bit from being raised over my head for so long. *Why can't this just be easy?*

I came out, defeated, and plunked down on the couch.

"What's up?" Mike asked.

"It's not working!" I said a little louder than I'd intended. "I've tried egg whites, glue sticks, liquid glue, and teasing it. I've already washed my hair twice, and I am cold and tired and hungry." I sounded like an angry six-year old. I hate when I sound like that.

Mike grabbed his computer. He typed away and then said, "Superstore is open for another twenty minutes. Let's go buy gel and hairspray."

I looked at him. It was an eighteen-minute drive. We would have about one minute to spare. We jumped up, ran out the door, and sped off down the highway as quickly as we could. We got there and I realized I was still in my bathrobe and my hair looked ridiculous. Mike quickly assessed me and just got out of the car. He knew I wasn't going in. After a few minutes he came back out and plopped the goods on my lap: super-hold hair gel and dynamo hairspray, twenty-four-hour hold. "Try this," he said.

We drove home and I got in the shower again. I was getting very tired. Between Maddie's birthday celebration and the hair chopping ceremony, this had been a big day. I grabbed the gel and blobbed it in. I blow-dried it. And, it fell flat. I laid on my side in bed and got Mike to blow-dry it again after I had thoroughly saturated it with the stinky hairspray. Again, nothing. "How the hell did Darlene *do this*?" I yelled. Hers was sheer perfection.

I started digging through my craft box once more and found a bottle of pink acrylic paint. It was about fifteen years old from when the kids were doing Easter crafts. I squeezed the bottle and a ton of it landed in my palm. I saw that it was full of dried bits and smelled awful, like a dead fish. I clasped my palms together, squishing the smelly paint back and forth, breaking down the larger chunks, and put it all in my hair with the dried, sticky hair-spray and gel. I styled it and it actually looked very cool, but I was bitterly disappointed that I couldn't get the mohawk up and running. Worst of all, we would be leaving at six a.m. and I had to sleep with this stinky mess on my head.

Mike could tell I was disappointed, this one bit of joy before chemo now a fail. I was planning on posting a pic of me heading into the Cancer

Centre all punked up with my hair done, pink poncho, boxing gloves, and pink camouflage leggings. I couldn't get this idea out of my mind. "Look," he said. "I know a guy. I bet he can superimpose a mohawk on a photo of you. Want me to ask him?"

"Yes please," I replied somewhat dejectedly but also feeling, as always, so very grateful for my incredibly supportive husband.

"Okay, go take a few selfies and I will send them off."

And so, I took selfies, tons of them, trying to get the right smile, the right lighting, the right angle, the right pose. It was a real challenge trying to get an authentic picture, given I was about to embark on a chemo journey in less than twelve hours. My mohawk fail was a big disappointment, and I tried hard to hide my fatigue and emotions. I felt like a phony as I smiled brightly, making my eyes excited. My eyes don't lie and I don't have much of a poker face. The hair situation with the fake mohawk was as if I'd desperately wanted the star role and ended up as the understudy, trying to be happy about it. I sent the pics to Mike who sent them to his good friend Steve, and half an hour later, the punk rocker version of me was created. I LOVED it. I looked wild. I was sporting a black leather jacket, crazy piercings, and a hot-pink mohawk that was sky-high. I waited until the next morning and promptly posted it.

Now, those who know me recognized that this wasn't actually my own hair, but those who hadn't seen me in a while thought it likely was. I felt a little awkward about it and had intended to explain the situation later but soon forgot all about the pic as the chemo began and I stepped headfirst into an unimaginably horrendous new battle.

24

CHEMO ROUND #1

Early the next morning, after I had posted the pic of me in my leather jacket with the pink mohawk, Mike and I began the journey into town. I kept checking my phone to see if any early risers had read my post yet.

Social Media Post #5
March 20

Chemo day, folks! Wish me luck.
See my "hair chopping" video in the comments section.

I was still disappointed that my planned mohawk hadn't turned out but was also quite pleased that the created one was almost bang-on to what I'd been attempting. I loved the picture; it was still my face, and I had finally managed, after many attempts, to capture the true essence of me. The hot-pink, sky-high mohawk definitely was an eye-catcher for scrollers. Already there were comments coming in, wishing me luck.

As we drove along on that dark, windy road, I silently prayed almost the whole way. *Please, dear God, let this go well. Please give me confidence. Please don't let me react to the chemo. Please allow my body to accept the chemo as a helpful medicine and not an evil, toxic poison.* On and on I continued, silently focusing on what I needed and what I was worried about. It takes great courage to start chemo, and I was wishing we lived a lot closer so I didn't have to travel for forty-five minutes feeling so worried and worked up.

I had hardly slept the night before. In addition to being incredibly anxious, my head was so darn itchy and full of paint, gel, and "hard as a rock" hairspray, that even if my mind had been calm, I could not get comfortable enough to actually sleep. I knew it was not good to start the day off feeling exhausted.

Trying to remain in control and not fly off into a full-fledged panic took a lot of focus and energy. It's hard being a grown-up and facing things you don't want to face, or to be clear, when you're completely terrified, forcing yourself to do what you don't want to do. In this battle I needed to be brave for my kids and my husband. I needed to show them I was strong, so that they could be strong in their own lives when they needed to be. I needed to show my husband that I could get through this, so he knew he had a partner who was his equal, just as tough. I wanted us to be side by side; I didn't want to be behind him as he dragged me into the ring of fire. I wanted to step in all on my own, to be a leader. So I told myself to move forward and to brace myself for the hit.

At last, we arrived. We parked and made the walk up to the front doors of the hospital, then past the security guards and down the long corridor of the Cancer Centre toward the elevators. Mike pushed the elevator button, and I nervously waited for it to arrive. The building was very old, and both things and people moved quite slowly. Finally, the doors opened and we squeezed in with many others, all masked and looking worn-out. We arrived to our floor and my heart resumed its pounding.

I entered the chemo center feeling extremely nervous and filled with incredible dread. There was a desk immediately off the elevator; I waited there as the receptionist typed away. When she finally looked up at me, I smiled, greeting her. "Good morning, I am Andrea Ritcey. I am here for chemo."

"Okay," she replied, without any further instruction. I stood there waiting for her to say something more, like "Take a seat," "Come this way," "Sign this document promising you won't sue us when you grow a third nipple and your skin turns green"—anything at all would have been helpful.

I waited another moment and then decided to add, "It's my first day. I'm not sure what to do."

She said, "I'm printing off some papers for you of upcoming appointments, and then you can have a seat."

I took the papers and looked around. "Uh, where are the seats?" I felt like she could have helped a bit more before I had to ask these questions.

Without looking up, she mumbled, "Around the corner."

There were a few different corners, actually, as we were in the centre point of a hexagon, but I nosed around and ultimately found the area that looked like it was meant for us.

Several other people were there with partners, all either bald, thin, puffy-faced, or slumping over, which confirmed to me that this was indeed the chemo waiting room. So I lugged my heavy bag over to an empty chair and sat there, now feeling a little foolish with my pink painted half-mohawk filled with hairspray and gunk and a suitcase-sized bag. I had packed a prayer shawl, my two snugglies from Annie and Maddie, my fleece blanket from Janet, plenty of snacks, a water bottle, my slippers, my phone charger, my ear phones, my computer, my computer charger, my Sudoku puzzle, pens and pencils, some colouring books, and some gum. I had no idea what was provided or what I would feel like doing, so I brought it all.

Right on the nose of my appointment time, a nurse called my name. She was tall and young and smiled warmly. "Come this way," she said. I was so very grateful for Mike; he had offered to come to every appointment and every chemo session. I felt helpless and scared, and he gave me much security. He grabbed my heavy bag and we walked down a long hall. The nurse brought us to a large, open room where there were about ten green La-Z-Boy chairs. Several people were already getting set up with IVs. "This is your spot for the day," she said pointing to the middle chair, and so I carefully sat in "my" chair. It was fairly comfortable. Mike's chair was wooden and as hard as a rock, which ultimately wreaked havoc on his back.

My nurse brought over a vitals machine and explained that they checked everything each time before they began the IVs, saline and chemo. My heart rate was 160. "Are you nervous?" she asked, looking concerned as she read the numbers. *Of course I'm nervous*, I thought. *Wouldn't you be?* But what could I say? *Yeah, lady, I'm terrified. I want to run out of here as fast as I can and never look back.*

"A little," I simply said, trying to play it cool. But my heart rate proved otherwise, and there was no getting around those numbers. My blood pressure was 150 over 112.

"Do you normally have high blood pressure?" she asked. I did normally, yes. And I took medication for it every day, but these numbers were not my normal, even with the medication. I explained all of this and she took notes. Then she reviewed my history of medications and asked if I had any drug allergies. My list is extensive and it took several minutes to get them all notated.

"Are you okay with needles?" she asked.

This time Mike made a sound—he sort of grunted. She looked up at him.

"*She* doesn't have a hard time with needles," he explained, "but *people* have a hard time getting them *in* her."

"Oh," said the nurse. "Well, we get two attempts and then we get another person."

"It's okay, I drank a ton of water yesterday; my veins should be primed and ready to go!" I tried to trick myself into feeling more confident than I was.

So, she got her things and began the search for a vein. The usual happened; she spent several minutes looking, tapping my arm, tightening the tourniquet, and struggling to find a good one. I nervously glanced around the room and saw that every other person was now settled in and happily "chemo-ing" away.

"Okay, I think I found one," she said.

I looked at Mike and he reached for my hand and gave it a squeeze. This was the first time he had witnessed the needle struggles I go through.

She poked, missed the vein, dug around, and retracted. "Sorry about that. Your veins are very tiny, and they keep moving."

I took in a deep breath and just waited. She tried again, and of course, was unsuccessful. My lip started quivering and Mike squeezed my hand harder. Another nurse came over and tried her hand at it; she too could not get the needle in. I just sat there, smiling away, but inside I felt so very defeated on this, my first day, and the first of many more chemo days to come.

"Have you considered a port?" nurse #2 asked.

My heart plunged. "Nope. Not at all." The idea of a port horrified me. I had heard awful stories of skin growing over, of them getting infected, of how they were sore and itchy and red and people struggled with them. If my skin wasn't so fair and delicate, perhaps I would go for it.

She too tried a second time and was unsuccessful. "I'm going to get Kailee." She smiled. "She's the best one here."

Kailee came over and in one swift move, got it in the side of my hand. "There you go. It's not great but it will do the job."

In my readings I learned that you can get chemo burns if the needle isn't perfectly placed. "Are you sure it's good?" I asked, trying hard not to cry. I was so scared.

"I think so. Here, let me double-check." She moved it a bit, and it pinched. "I think we're good to go."

We were now an hour into the appointment time and only just starting the fluids. She brought some bags over and checked the ID band on my wrist. She read the numbers on my arm and the numbers on the bag. She began with a saline drip. (Saline is used to prevent nephrotoxicity, a rapid decline in the kidney function, and to increase renal blood flow. I happen to have a ten-centimetre cyst on my kidney, so the fact that they could go downhill fast really freaked me out. Kidney failure can be fatal.)

The saline drip took about thirty minutes and I watched as my hand slowly puffed up, turned cold, and became sore. I asked the nurse if that was normal. "Hmm," she said, looking a little miffed. "Not really. I mean, it does happen, but it shouldn't." She ended up returning every ten minutes to see how I was doing. After the saline drip, they started the Paclitaxel. The nurse read the numbers again on my wrist and then on the bag. Then another nurse was called over to double-check the numbers. I liked how careful and thorough they were. No mix-ups at the Dickson Centre today!

She hooked the IV line up to the chemo and explained that I was to make certain to tell her if I felt any reaction at all—sore stomach, itchy tongue, etc. I nodded. I felt a little like when you are clamped into a rickety old roller coaster and it's your last possible second to back out before facing imminent death. "And . . . here we go," she said while pressing buttons. She smiled warmly as she released the poison. I felt breathless and panicky as I watched it start. I was not sure if my body would react, I had so many allergies. Oddly, a minute after it started, I felt pain in my lower back. I mentioned this and the nurse and Mike both said it could just be the chair. Yes, I *had* ended up a little slumped and my feet were up, but it seemed odd to me that the pain in my back only started at the same time as the chemo.

It took a full four hours for the Paclitaxel to be fully delivered in me, and I spent the time on my phone reading wonderful, encouraging comments, trying to sleep, listening to music, and eating snacks. I was pleased to learn that snacks were provided, and I ate an egg sandwich and a banana. Because the IV needle ended up being placed in my hand instead of my arm, it prevented me from using the bathroom by myself or doing anything independently the entire day. Mike had to escort me to the bathroom four times, as the fluids all had to come out somehow. He had to hike my pants down, and hike them back up each and every time. I felt humiliated and embarrassed at my inability to even perform such a simple task.

We had now been at it for roughly six hours—from the hour prep to get the IV needle in; another hour prepping with saline, steroids, and various other fluids and some discussion; and then four more hours for the actual chemo—and we hadn't even started the second chemo drug. Eventually the nurses set up another saline drip and then started the Carboplatin. I had to sit in the chair for eight long hours that day. All in all, the procedures of the day went quite well, and I was relieved at how truly knowledgeable, kind, and efficient the nurses were in this unit. I was completely exhausted from the effort it took to be brave. I was mentally drained trying to keep all of the new information sorted out in my head—the process was all so new.

Toward the end of the day, a man looking like he was physically in very rough shape walked across the floor to the nurse's station. The staff announced that he had completed his chemo treatments. He looked so very happy but yet so very sick. They handed him a big brass bell. "What is he doing?" I whispered to Mike.

"I think he's supposed to ring the bell because he's done the treatments," he whispered back.

"What? That's so cool!" I exclaimed, totally intrigued.

A nurse introduced him and announced that he had just completed nine rounds of chemo, and then, smiling a shy smile, the man weakly rang the bell. I was bursting with happiness for him, so I yelled a loud "Whoo hoo!" and, even though it hurt my puffy hand with the needle in it, I began clapping hard claps. I looked around. No one else was clapping. I was surprised by that. "Congratulations!" I yelled to him as enthusiastically as I could.

I was intrigued. I looked up the history on the bell and came across a poem by US rear admiral Irve Le Moyne:

Ringing Out

Ring this bell
Three times well
It's toll to clearly say,

My treatment's done
This course is run
And I am on my way!

When asked about his own cancer treatment back in 1996 and why he rang the bell, R.A. Le Moyne stated that when a job is done in the Navy, the tradition is to ring the bell. He brought a brass bell to his own last cancer treatment, rang it and then left it as a donation. They are now ringing bells all over the world to signify the job is done, the treatment complete. The ringing of the bell that day planted a seed for me and I began picturing a special ceremony and my own "ringing the bell" moment. I loved the whole idea of this.

Two more hours slowly passed and finally, we finished at six o'clock. The room was empty except for the two of us and the one last nurse remaining on staff. She came over and removed my IV.

"That was a long day," Mike said, stretching his back as he stood up. He had stayed by my side the entire day and was looking quite stiff. My back was full-on aching, and I was feeling heavy and tired.

We made the long drive home to "The Log," and Duey greeted us exuberantly. I met him at the door and then panicked as I didn't know if it was okay that he was licking me with the chemo in my body. I was told that no one could use my bathroom for the first few days and that I even had to put the lid down first before I flushed so that no water mixed with chemo pee would get on the seat, the floor or anywhere in contact with others. It was a lot to remember.

That evening I started feeling poorly; I was told I would have a rapid drop in white blood cells. It started with a headache. My temperature rose and I had chills. I started getting muscle aches. My face started swelling and was itchy and red. I followed the clear instructions on the papers and took all the anti-nauseates and steroids and pain meds. Mike helped me get set up in the main floor guest room as the bathroom was closer and the bed easier to get out of. The kitchen and main room were also on this floor, so I could avoid the extra effort of doing the stairs. I didn't want Duey sleeping on top of me, nor did I want him or Mike somehow being exposed to the chemo in me.

Mike and I spent the evening on the couch together and then I said goodnight, quite fearful of how the night would go. Heavily drugged, I managed to sleep through the wee hours, only getting up once to pee. But by early morning, I woke up quite miserable. My face was now completely flushed, quite swollen, and I had a full-body rash. The pain in my lower spine was shooting right down to my feet. I hobbled to the bathroom and dug around for my toothbrush.

All of a sudden I felt like I was going to faint. Dizzy and seeing black tunnels, I staggered back to bed. "Mike!" I called loudly, "I need you!" He came up right away and was surprised to see my red, swollen face and to learn how awful I felt. I was extremely short of breath and my heart rate soared to 180. We read the sheets, took the pills, and tried numerous things to help—heating pads, ice packs, morphine—but nothing helped at all. By lunchtime I was full-on squirming and moaning uncontrollably. I popped hydromorphone like it was sugar pills and tried calling the Cancer Centre. I could not get comfortable and couldn't stand it anymore. I suffered terribly. Boy oh boy, did I suffer. I suffered like that for two days straight, and it was all I could do to not lose my mind.

At forty-eight hours in, we decided I needed to go to emerg. We felt pretty strongly that the pain should not be this bad, and I needed something stronger to manage. We made the trip to emerg at four o'clock that afternoon. I made certain we brought my binder with all of my chemo info and made sure I had the special yellow card to fast-track past the non-cancer patients.

The drive in was insufferable, and I cried most of the way. Finally, we arrived and I got my yellow card out as soon as I got into the main lobby of the hospital. Mike grabbed a wheelchair for me as I couldn't walk. I was in so much pain and so ill that I was shaking uncontrollably. I showed the check-in lady my yellow card. Not much was said about it. I was then directed to sit in another space right in the main emerg area, and we were not triaged until a full hour after arriving.

The wait in that fully packed room with everyone all around me was dreadful. I was immune compromised and yet I had people coughing all around me. I was in so much pain I was unable to remain quiet, and I whimpered and rocked back and forth in my wheelchair feeling like I was going to die. After we were triaged and I had shown my yellow card again, we were moved behind the main area and there I remained for another three miserable hours. I squirmed and rocked and whimpered and cried out in pain and tried my best not to make a scene. It was the most trying of nights, and no one was helping us. In the initial consult prior to chemo I'd been assured that I would be seen within thirty minutes of arrival, and yet unbelievably, four long, painstaking, miserable hours went by. I kept asking nurses who walked by if someone could get me some pain management and no one did.

I was basically treated no differently than any other patient there, even though cancer patients are supposed to be top priority. Ridiculously, we waited for a total of eight hours and still were not taken to a room or seen by a doctor. It is impossible to relay the severe amount of pain I was in. Unless you have walked this very same path, there are simply no words to describe how truly dire my situation was. The pain was at a ten on a scale of one to ten. If pain alone could kill you, I would be dead. I was not able to do anything but fight with all my might to keep from passing out, fearful I would have a heart attack or a full-blown mental breakdown. It was the most extended length of time I have ever dealt with severe pain, without any pain meds. I learned many months later that reactions like mine are documented as rare cases; only 1-3 percent of the population reacts as severely to the chemo as I did.

It got to the point that I was going to lie on the filthy hospital floor as I could not manage to stay upright any longer. We decided to go home as I was no longer able to remain lucid and desperately wanted my own bed. Surely to goodness this intense pain would pass soon, we naively reasoned—it had been fifty-six hours so far. Mike wheeled me out to the car. I was crying uncontrollably, my face shoved in my sweater so as not to upset the other patients. I struggled to get my legs in the car as they had lost all feeling and I couldn't get my brain to send the message to lift them up. It was midnight and raining hard. As I finally got tucked into the car, a nurse ran out to us and said, "Why are you leaving? You shouldn't go home."

I looked at her, still sobbing. "I have cancer! I'm having a severe reaction to the chemo and need help and pain meds and we've been here for eight hours! I cannot physically sit up in that wheelchair any longer. I *have* to go home." With that, Mike pulled away and we headed home.

I was so desperate for sleep that I extended the car seat and attempted to stretch out, even though the severe spinal pain was keeping me curled in a ball. From the drive in, the wait, and the drive out, it was another ten hours with no medical intervention. Never in my life have I had to endure so much and I was completely spent.

I continued to suffer horribly the next several days with no relief in sight. I rolled around in my bed as a coping mechanism, unable to lie still from the deepest bone pain I have ever experienced in my life. My pain was still intensely acute and still at a full, rolling ten. I alternated between being in a tight, fetal ball (this was only seven weeks' post-hysterectomy, and I was nowhere near comfortable in the abdominal area but the severe pain forced me to curl up) and fully squirming, rocking and panting as I tried my hardest to get control of the pain.

By Saturday, after taking Tylenol with codeine, Advil, Aleve, doubling up on the hydromorphone, and trying many other things, the pain had still not gotten any better and we decided to make the long trek in again. This was now five full days without any reprieve from severe and debilitating spinal nerve pain and deep, full-body muscle and bone pain. On the way to the hospital my heart was acting up so much that I debated calling 911 to get an ambulance to meet us along the road. I knew this was not a good plan since the province's ambulance service is so flawed.

"Mike," I moaned, almost inaudibly.

"Yes?"

"Are you up to date on your life-saving skills?" Mike is a former lifeguard and has saved people in the past.

"I think so, yes. Why?"

"My heart is acting very funny, and I am having severe chest pain. I think I might possibly have a heart attack, and I want you to know that, in case I slump over."

He looked hard at me, assessing what to do, and we both realized the answer was to keep driving as fast as possible.

Emerg was packed full of the usual Saturday night specials and was busy and loud. At one point I started shaking so hard that my hands went completely numb and they froze in a lobster claw position. Thankfully I was alert enough to know I suddenly and urgently needed to use the bathroom. I was again in a wheelchair and knew I couldn't get there fast enough by myself. In a panic, I moaned to Mike, "I need you to get me to a bathroom as soon as you can. I can't hold on. I'm about to lose all control from both ends."

Mike asked the security guard where to take me and then began racing down the hallway as fast as he could. "Hang on. Hang on!" he encouraged and pleaded, as I panted and rocked, trying not to poop, pee, or pass out. I was seeing spiralling black tunnels again and losing my vision. My severe pain was causing me to faint. Mike got me to the bathroom and I got on the toilet just as my body violently expelled horrible gas, poop, and pee. I made a mess in that bathroom yet my hands were still frozen in lobster claws and I couldn't grasp the toilet paper. My hands were useless. I had to yell for Mike to come in and get me some toilet paper and I did my best to clean myself up while still panting and seeing black tunnels.

Incredibly, we waited for two hours before they finally called me for blood work, even though I should have been seen right away. I tried to walk the five feet from the wheelchair to the blood collection La-Z-Boy, and I felt my legs give out. I could not raise my feet, and I felt severe pain in my spine, cutting off the nerve pathways to my legs. I fell into the La-Z-Boy and waited for twenty more minutes.

"You can't sit there," a nurse firmly announced as she came over.

I replied, "They called me for blood work; I *am* supposed to sit here."

It was obvious I was critically ill and yet the nurse made me get up and move. I slumped and dragged myself back to my wheelchair. Then they called my name again and once more I dragged and crawled as best I could to the chair. The fact that my legs were not working was very scary in and of itself. My hands were still frozen in lobster claws while the technician tried to pull them apart to prep me for blood work.

She poked me four times, twice trying to get the blood work and twice to get an IV in. They were going to run a CT scan with dye in my lumbar region to see why I was in so much pain. Ultimately we were there for another six-hour visit, with no answers and no extra pain management.

We returned home and in the next several days I had three fainting spells. When I showered, my blood pressure dropped so low that I would stagger out in the middle of my efforts, soaking wet and freezing cold, panting and stumbling to the nearest bed. I could not stand or walk without collapsing, so ultimately no showers were to be had. Baths were virtually impossible as I got so dizzy going from a laying position to an upright one to get out of the tub that again, that I was left stumbling, soaking wet and crashing face down on the nearest bed, dripping water all over the bedding, seeing tunnels and panting hard.

I continued to have debilitating back pain and the morphine didn't come close to touching any of the pain. On day twelve, as promised, my hair started falling out. The hair loss included eyelashes, eyebrows, underarm, pubic, and leg hair.

To make matters even worse, diarrhea began and was miserably painful due to my back end being still very much destroyed and the huge external hemorrhoid was still flaring from the clay-baby episode just seven weeks before. During this time Mike continued to work from home and brought me soups, water, toast, medicine, pain meds, and looked after everything I needed. Boy oh boy I sure kept him busy; he was exceptionally patient. I had developed neuropathy in my fingers and toes and therefore could not hold my toothbrush or button up buttons or even hold a drinking glass. We were warned in chemo that my electrolytes would be affected. Indeed they were as I was left feeling even weaker with low sodium, magnesium, potassium, and calcium. My heart rhythm changed and was constantly fluttering, and I had severe chest pains. I knew my lungs likely had damage as well; I was left constantly coughing and breathless.

This was, with absolutely no exception, the worst moments in all of my entire life; the fact that I was expected to go through this five more times was both terrifying and totally mind bending.

25

LARA AND THE GREAT SURPRISE

Miraculously, by day thirteen the pain had noticeably lessened. That change in itself brought me enormous relief physically and mentally. I had finally come out the other side of an extremely intense two weeks. I had been thoroughly challenged both psychologically and physically; it was relentless, exhausting, and unbearable.

My bedsheets at this point needed a thorough washing as they had sweat, leaks, and various food spills from me eating the majority of my meals in bed. Dog fur and sand also coloured this mixed array, from our beloved Duey. He refused to leave my side and insisted on climbing into bed with me even in the little guest room. Stains from creams like Voltaren and cannabis oil had absorbed and marked the sheets, and yet it was too much effort to even think of stripping the bed. Finally, I had had enough and rose to attempt some very light cleaning. I pulled one sheet corner off of the bed and was disappointed to realize the task seemed incredibly demanding.

The effort it took sent me crashing face first on the mattress. Panting with a racing heart, I got up and tried again. I stepped over the heavy quilt and pillows now on the floor and began pulling at the next corner. That was it. I couldn't even take a dirty sheet off of my own bed. I laid down to catch my breath and promptly fell asleep sideways, sheets, blankets, and pillows strewn all around me on the bed and on the floor, looking much like a bomb had gone off.

Mike came up the stairs a while later and gently shook me awake to make sure I was okay. "Can you please strip the bed for me?" I asked, sounding just so feeble.

"Of course!" he answered and got to it right away. I piled my comforter back on and curled right back up to sleep. Looking back, that moment was very telling; from then on I would never take for granted a single thing my body can do, even changing the sheets.

As the day wore on, I was amazed that I was able to manage with just the Tylenol with codeine and heating pads. I still had very little energy, but I was able to sit in the living room for a short while before having to go back to bed.

By day fourteen I felt well enough to consider having a very short visit from a dear friend the following day. The plan was she would come for one hour. I would lay on the couch and be loaded up on meds and just remain there. No walking to the door to greet her, no making tea. That evening, however, the emotional trauma hit me as I started processing my severely damaged, weakened state, the past several months of physical pain from both the hysterectomy and the very bad chemo reaction. Ominous thoughts of the long road ahead completely overwhelmed me. Again I felt scared and completely defeated. I began crying and confessed to Mike that I was terrified to start another round of chemo in little over a week. I laid on the couch with my head in his lap, exhausted, scared, sad, and sore. I fell asleep with him stroking the last bits of my hair.

The next morning, I woke up with a headache. I still felt weak and exhausted, and deeply, darkly sad. I cancelled my visit with my dear friend. At lunchtime, my sister wanted to FaceTime me. She had had a migraine the day before and was unable to FaceTime me then, so I was looking forward to her sweet face and cheery smile. She told me she would connect with me at one p.m., and, exactly at 1:00, my phone rang.

Lara looked to be outside—I could see trees all around her. She had a very large grin on her face as I said hello. "Wow, Andrea, your place looks amazing!" she said exuberantly. I was confused. I looked past her face on the screen to the scene behind her. It *did* look like our place, but that didn't make any sense at all. I was exhausted and heavily drugged. I could see a familiar coastline behind her. She grinned away, watching my reaction. I was confused and reasoned that Mike had somehow superimposed a green screen behind her to make it look like she was here. He is an IT specialist, so I wouldn't put it past him to get creative.

Lara began walking around, and I could see more of my property over her shoulder. I was even more confused. *Is she here? This can't be. She lives in California.* She started laughing some more and said, "I absolutely love Duey, by the way. We are already friends." And then I heard steps on my front porch. *What? She IS here!* I jumped out of bed and raced across the living room, regretting my haste instantly as pain shot through my entire body. My heart felt ready to explode and I was badly out of breath. I yanked open the heavy front door and to my complete and utter shock and sheer joy, I saw her, standing there, all smiles.

"Lara!" I screeched, and leapt into her arms. I broke down in body-wracking sobs and heavy, fast-flowing tears. I held on to her with all my might and squeezed her so hard our bodies felt like one. She held me in her arms just as tightly and squeezed me just as hard. It felt like an eternity of lifetimes passing between us as we stood there, crying and embracing, both of us immensely relieved to be together and that we had made it through our surgeries and my first round of chemo. The pure energy of love and joy that passed between us made our hearts feel like two magnets stuck together. It is tough to describe that heart connection in words, but it was powerful, solid, and direct.

I am sure Lara was not expecting to be greeted by me in this way, jumping on her and heavily sobbing, and I was equally not expecting to feel the true magnitude of our exchange. My emotions were all over the place, and I was incredibly fragile with all that I had been through. Her emotions were also fragile; she had been worried and scared for me for four months, fresh out of her own hysterectomy, and wiped from travelling across the country when she should've still been in bed. She told me she had felt helpless living across the country, unable to hug me, see me, check in with me as I processed my cancer.

Duey started barking in excitement, and I released the hug and stared at my sister in disbelief. "Wha? How? Oh my gosh, I can't even talk! Is this real? Am I dreaming?"

She smiled the biggest smile I have ever seen from her and looked me square in the eye. "This is real. I am here." She rubbed my back.

"Wow!" I yelled, with utter joy. "Wow. Wow. Wow!"

She laughed and said, "I'm here for three whole weeks!"

"You are?" I was incredulous.

"Yup. I want to make sure my baby sissy is okay!" She glanced around and looked over my shoulder at our log home, seeing it for the very first time. "Wow! This place is fabulous! Now, give me a tour!"

Mike stood there grinning.

"Did you know about this?" I asked, still amazed.

"Of course!" he said, happy the surprise had come off so perfectly. They had planned it weeks ago. As it turned out, Lara didn't actually have a migraine yesterday, she was en route. At this point, she was only five weeks' post-hysterectomy, and yet she had flown across the continent to see me. I was in awe at how well she looked.

As my adrenalin settled, weakness registered in the front of my brain. Aware of my acute pain once more, I suddenly needed to sit down and catch my breath.

Lara was amazed by our beautiful home. "Oh my gosh. This is spectacular!" she sang. She walked across to the windows and looked at the ocean crashing below on the rocky coastline. "Andrea! This is the most magical place you could possibly have. It's the perfect space for you on this journey!"

After a while she became tired herself, and I said, "Let's keep talking, but can we get in my bed? I really need to lie down." She got right under the covers with me and we lay there, spooning, my arms wrapped around her. We giggled and talked and fell asleep.

About two hours later, we woke up from our glorious nap. It was a turning point in our relationship.

"We finally shared a bed without fighting!" I proclaimed, laughing.

"Now you don't have to sleep in the baby crib!" she exclaimed happily and we laughed even more. We reminisced about the fact that when we were children, forced to share a double bed at Nana's house, we always ended up kicking and fighting. Ultimately I would get kicked out of the bed and would have to sleep in the leftover baby crib that Nana had kept in the office. I'd sleep in it with my legs all bunched up as I was far too big for it. I can remember wondering why I always had to get the crib and Lara would have the entire double bed.

The next morning, Lara woke up and went to the kitchen. I was feeling poorly again; the night before had taken a lot out of me, energy-wise. Mike was up already making coffee and eggs, and Lara started planning our meals for the day with nourishment and sustenance from the cookbooks she had sent a few weeks earlier. Still unable to stand for any length of time, I decided to head on over to the couch, and Lara followed with coffee in hand. Duey followed as well. Although this unfamiliar person seemed quite similar to me, his beloved mama, Duey was not ready to let his guard down. I plunked myself down on the couch, and Lara started to step in to join me. Duey, who at this point had never been on the couch in our new home, stepped quickly past her, hip checking her swiftly aside as he moved. In one deft jump, he gracefully leapt from beside Lara, high into the air, over our large coffee table, and onto the couch beside me. He somehow managed to turn his giant body adeptly around in the tight diameter of the couch, and he firmly sat on his bottom. Not yet finished, he fully extended his chest and looked quite tall, very dignified, and intentionally, yet silently, communicating a poignant message to my sister.

"Duey!" I cried. "What are you doing?"

With not so much as a sound, he had protected me and effectively got the point across that he would be the one sitting next to me this morning and absolutely no one else. He had never done this before. After she regained her balance from the hip-check, Lara cracked up laughing.

"Well, okay. Thanks, Duey! I guess I won't be sitting next to Andrea right now!"

Duey watched her carefully as she took a side seat. He didn't look scary, just stubborn, like, "Just try and move me. I'm not leaving Mama's side." He knew his weight.

I was impressed by him. Lara had always raised golden retrievers and was completely fascinated by this instinct of his. She observed keenly my relationship with Duey and his with me. She remarked how intuitive he was and how incredibly well I knew my dog. Once again I said a silent thank you to the universe for giving me the gift of time with this beautiful creature. Mastiffs truly are the most incredible of dogs. They have existed for over 2,500 years, all the while studying their human's behavior and are genius at reading body language and silently protecting them.

Within the next two days, Duey came to really trust and enjoy Lara and ultimately showed his gratitude. We'd been watching a movie and he decided once again to get up on the couch. He pushed his way between us, but this time, to our surprise, he plunked his head down right over Lara's heart and promptly fell asleep, snoring heavily. We both looked at each other. Simultaneously we crooned, "Aw!" and I could tell Lara was quite flattered. I truly think it was Duey's way of showing he not only accepted her, but was also thankful for her care with me.

And Duey was right. She did take really great care of me during our time together. She insisted I drink a lot more water, she made me tea, salads, wonderful meals and poured over the cookbooks to ensure I was getting all the nutrients I needed and, she gave Mike a much needed break so he could focus more on his work. By about day sixteen post-chemo, I was feeling well enough that I could sit at the dinner table for ten minutes to eat a meal.

Feeling well enough also meant I was able to start acting like my old self . . . a little.

26

CALL ME CRAZY OR CALL ME DESPERATE OR MAYBE JUST CALL ME A COMEDIAN

In hindsight, maybe it wasn't such a great idea to duct-tape my head. Yes, we had cut my hair short, almost to the scalp, but it was still bothering me. Although the hair that was left now from the chemo was just short spiky bits that would fall in my eyes, my nose, my mouth, the back of my neck, and all over my sweaters. I would wake up regularly with a mess of orangey-peach fuzz all over my pillow, and while in the shower, I had to deal with large clumps of those fuzzies stuck on my hands, all over the soap, and clogging the drain. I would use my towel to dry off my scalp and then my body, only to have those short, annoying spikes transfer in the towel from my scalp to my still-damp skin; those hairs then found themselves on and in all other parts of me. Enough was enough, and I couldn't be bald fast enough.

"Mike!" I yelled. "Get the duct tape!"

Lara and Mike had been drinking a glass of wine in the kitchen, and I was glad the two of them were spending some quality time together. In the past, the three of us discovered we were a funny dynamic whereby I often ended up feeling a little rebellious, daring, wild. I'm not sure what possessed me to think it was a good idea to duct-tape my head, but at this point, I had been in the same small guest room, lying in bed, looking at the same four walls for the better half of almost three months. I was feeling both heavily depressed and physically miserable. I was desperate for something to laugh about.

Mike came to see what was going on. He held his glass of red wine in one hand and leaned up against the door frame looking down at me. "Did I hear you say you needed duct tape?" he asked.

My sister had followed behind and was looking over his shoulder. "Duct tape?" she repeated.

I was lying on my stomach, my feet up behind me swinging away, trying to manage more pain and boredom. "Yes," I mumbled, my face in my pillow. "Duct tape."

"Whatever for?" Mike asked.

"To get the rest of my stupid hair off. It's driving me crazy!" I waited for their response.

"Okay," Mike said, and started to turn around.

"Wait, what?" Lara said, suspending the plan. "Andrea, let me get this straight. You want to duct-tape your head?" She was looking at me with fascination and confusion; concerned yet laughing in amazement that I was actually proposing this crazy idea.

"Yup," I replied.

"Okay, Andrea, you can't duct-tape your head. Won't that hurt?"

I heard love and unease in her voice, paired with amusement.

"I don't care; my hair is driving me crazy!" I announced again. I mean really, it wasn't that insane an idea. The duct tape wasn't going directly on my skin; it was for all the short, spiky bits that kept rubbing off with every move I made.

Mike arrived back with the duct tape. "Where do you want me to tape?" he asked, ready and confident in my plan.

"Okay, slow down. Let's talk about this," Lara interjected as Mike looked for the starting point on the roll.

Lara sat beside me on the bed, and I explained to her how I didn't think it would be too bad and carefully reasoned with her. Mike agreed and yanked hard on the tape. It made the familiar ripping noise as it unstuck itself from the roll. He gently placed it right above my ears and started carefully winding it around my head. Lara, now seeing that the two of us were actually just that nutty to pull such a stunt shrieked in disbelief, her wine sloshing precariously in the glass.

"You're serious. You're really doing this! Oh my gosh, Mike. Stop, you're going to hurt her!" She was laughing hard at this point. I heard him reassure her I would be okay, and then he slowly ripped off the end of the tape from the roll. He started on to the other side, and I started giggling. I loved this moment—my sister laughing at such a ridiculous interaction between husband and wife. "I can't believe you guys. You're both completely nuts!"

"Well, ya gotta have some fun in life, right?" Mike said, laughing as he worked. "And, hey, what else are we gonna do on a Tuesday night?" Mike laughed even harder as he ripped the second piece off the roll.

"Ha! You two are hilarious!" Lara said, nodding.

"Ready?" Mike asked.

"Ready," was my heavily muffled response, face still in the pillow.

Mike placed his hand on my back, and with his other hand I could feel his knuckles dig under the first piece of tape. *Rriiiiippp!* I felt it pull the hairs out.

"Oh my gosh!" Lara shrieked with more laughter. "Are you okay, Andrea?"

With physical comedy, timing is everything. So naturally, I gave a worrisome, quiet pause, building the suspense, before I boldly stuck my head up and yelled, "Wee haw! Do it again!"

My sister completely lost it at that point, gales of laughter ringing out, as Mike shook the sticky, hairy tape off of his fingers. He dug in for number two and yanked a little faster, a little harder, and it only hurt just a wee bit. My face bounced back into the pillow. "Ow!" I yelled. "Okay, that's good, that's good!"

Mike was laughing even harder now, and I too was laughing. Lara was completely bent over, howling.

"Lara, did ya ever think you were going to come home to see this?" I yelled up to her, still muffled.

"Oh my good God, no!" She had her hand on my shoulder. "You two are the absolute best. You're just so . . . outrageous!" She was clearly pleased to witness our crazy relationship. She started to settle then as the dire reality hit us for the millionth time. She was looking at me now with sadness, as I lay there, almost completely bald, and starting to feel the fatigue from the effort of our escapade. My laughter had exhausted me—such a contrast to mere moments before.

I moved my hands up and around my pillow, reaching for the sides of my head. My fingertips searching for confirmation that the job had indeed been done. With my arms no longer supporting my torso, my face sunk deeper into the pillow. My scalp felt sticky, but the hair was undeniably gone. "Okay, that's good. I better leave the rest, in case what we did destroyed the hair follicle and it doesn't grow back." I patted the sides again; it felt a lot better. Lara and Mike cleaned up the tape, the wine droplets on the floor, and the spriglets of hair everywhere. I flipped my pillow over as it was covered in drool from my laughter, and I promptly fell asleep.

Two days later the rest of my spriggly-bits fell out anyway, and I officially reached the "bald as an egg" status that Dr. Scott had so assuredly promised.

Social Media Post #6
April 10

> Well folks, tomorrow is chemo Round #2. I'm feeling a bit of dread. My first round (March 20th) was extremely challenging. I had full-blown reactions with two trips to Emergency (a total of 14 horrific hours waiting there to be assessed), two blood draws, a CT scan, three fainting spells, a full-body rash, and severe itch for three days, debilitating back and bone pain that caused brief loss of usage in hands, and the loss of use of feet and legs (morphine didn't even touch the pain!), fevers, swollen red face, and a complete loss of hair. I'm now completely bald. Chemo is a rough, rough go. I'm floored at the strength of chemo warriors / cancer survivors. I pray tomorrow will go smoothly. (Including, perhaps, more success this time with getting the IV in . . . 4 attempts last

time and success on try #5, ugh). I just wanted to pop on here and give the update, soo there it is. ♡ I'm so, soo, soo grateful for all the prayers and support. Perhaps tomorrow if people could say a little prayer for me that my body will accept the miracle juice gracefully and easily, and a smoother round for Chemo #2, maybe the universe will come through for me!

Love you all soo much, my dear peeps. ☺

Within mere minutes, my ever faithful media community of friends started sending me the kindest messages. "You got this!" "You can do it!" "You are so brave!" "Sending prayers," et cetera. It was quite honestly exactly what I needed to read. It made me gain confidence and mental strength. Again, the power of the written word.

27
CHEMO ROUND #2 AND THE CHEMICAL WIZARDS

I took a close-up picture of my bubble-gum pink boxing gloves, and underneath the picture I simply captioned:

Social Media Post #7
April 11

Round 2. Bing! Bing!

Again, we drove in at the crack of dawn from our home in the little village on the ocean. Traffic was never an issue in this part of the region, but once we hit Halifax it was another story; bumper-to-bumper traffic and endless red lights. I was keen to arrive at the Cancer Centre several minutes early, basically to calm my nerves and to collect myself.

At first it was a quiet drive in with very little to say as I had slept poorly and was feeling jittery. Mike, as usual, sensed this and placed his hand on my knee as he drove. Outwardly, he was Mr. King of Relaxed.

We arrived at the Cancer Centre quite rattled, as on the last fifteen minutes of our drive we had three near accidents, all of which were very close calls. I felt like we were in a video game, dodging, swerving, honking, and yelling. My adrenalin was pumping and my nerves were shot; not a great way to start the chemo process.

Mike parked, I brought in my much less packed bag, and we checked in. We then went to the now familiar waiting area. Eventually I heard my name called and I looked up. A short, friendly lady introduced herself (Mary, from Newfoundland), and off we went. I sat in the same ugly green chair and recognized some faces from three weeks prior. It's truly odd how you can fear something your whole life knowing that it is supposed to be awful and then you experience the treatment, have amazing nurses doing the chemo and then it becomes almost comforting when you return. "It's Get Better juice," I started telling myself, so I wouldn't go down endless rabbit holes about what was actually going in my body.

I told Nurse Mary about my troubles last time, the trips to emerg, the five pokes from three different nurses. She looked at me with kindness. "We will get this done with less than five, I promise."

I was about fifty-fifty on the believer scale but smiled at her and bravely said, "Okay. Let's go."

And, miraculously, she got the IV in on the first try!

"This is great, Mary! You've already made today much better than last time."

Into routine, she went about getting things ready. I was given the saline solution, a few other chemo-prep things, and then, about forty-five minutes in, we started the paclitaxel. Drip, drip, drip . . .

"Take your mask down, please, so I can see your face." Mary needed to see my lips in case there was swelling. *Was it just me or was I feeling rather odd?* She pulled up a stool. "Now, if you start to feel like you are getting a reaction, you need to tell me right away, okay?"

I was looking at her while she spoke but was not quite taking in what she said because my stomach had started to feel very, painfully weird. I was trying to focus on her. She started describing a little more about breathing issues and allergic reactions, and I knew it was important to listen. I was trying really hard to focus. I waited for her to finish as I didn't want to interrupt, but then I quickly started feeling this odd feeling of impending doom. I knew exactly what she was talking about, as I was experiencing everything she was describing as she was describing it. I should have said it a minute or two earlier, but had politely waited. Now it had evolved into a true emergency. I blurted out, "I'm not feeling well at all! I'm having a reaction!"

Instantly I could feel my heart racing more rapidly than it ever had before, and my body felt like I was on a circus ride, spinning faster and faster. I felt like I was plummeting to the ground from an airplane.

Super calm Mary jumped into action. "I need a vitals machine, stat!" she yelled. I was surprised at how loud she yelled it. Within seconds, three nurses raced over, expertly and hastily rolling the machines toward me.

I felt like I was about to pass out and I closed my eyes tight. My body was shutting down. I wasn't sure if they knew how quickly this was hitting me, but I needed to tell them and heard myself say, "Get going, ladies, I can't hold on much longer."

"She's really red," I heard Mike say from my left. He sounded concerned.

"Yes, that's her blood pressure shooting up," explained someone behind me.

I heard feet moving all around me, nimbly. I felt Mike take my hand as machines beeped faster. Someone else whipped my chair back and my feet went up.

"Do you have an epi pen?" I mumbled, barely conscious but still fighting.

"It's already going in," Mary replied, reassuringly.

I couldn't feel it so I managed to open my eyes a wee bit and saw Mary had a syringe attached to a tube, and her thumb was firmly pressing down on the top. Clear liquid was going into the IV line. I felt like I was going to lose consciousness. Everything started feeling maxed-out crazy, like I was going to die.

"She's still really flushed," Mike said, louder over the chaos.

"Yup, working on that. Her heart rate will go down in about thirty seconds," Mary said firmly.

I felt a cold cloth on my forehead and someone behind me started speaking really loudly. "How are you doing, Andrea? Can you hear me?"

"Yes," I croaked. I could barely speak. My throat was super dry and my tongue felt huge and swollen, like it was caught in a mouse trap. "I feel awful," I said. My chest pained badly and I struggled to breathe.

"You are going to be just fine," someone said. "Just focus on your breathing. Try and breathe slowly, in through your nose and out through your mouth."

I did this for several seconds and didn't get worse. After a few minutes of this, I started to come around. I opened my eyes then. Mike was staring at me, relieved. Someone else crossed over and approached me.

"Andrea, we are going to get an EKG of your heart to make sure you are doing okay, alright?"

I nodded. Mike squeezed my hand. I was completely in another world. My head felt like it was rolling around. "What just happened?" I asked, blinking and blurry. I had an awful taste in my mouth.

"You had a bit of a reaction there," Nurse Mary said. "But we gotcha. You just need a few minutes to recover."

"Am I allergic to the chemo?" I asked, secretly hoping that would be the end of it.

"Yes. You had a strong allergic reaction, but we will give you lots of Benadryl and we will get it in ya, don't you worry."

What? Had I heard her correctly? I am sure she saw the shock and worry cross my very unwell face.

"We can override the body's response to the chemo by giving you lots of Benadryl and steroids. We can adjust the speed of the drip and go extra slowly," she explained.

Oh my God, they're going to kill me, I thought. *This is nuts.*

I looked at Mike. He smiled at me and said, "You're okay. I'm here." He was trying to reassure me, but I've known him long enough to read that he too was worried.

"We got twenty-five mls in ya," I heard Mary say. "We've got 150 more to go."

I was terrified. I didn't understand how it was possible to trick the body and override the histamine reaction. Remaining in that chair and trusting the nurses took a huge amount of effort for me. And you know what? Miraculously, they managed to get the rest of the paclitaxel in. They indeed changed the drip speed to super slow, and then I had saline, and then more steroids. Then they started the carboplatin and I was extremely nervous again, afraid I would also have a bad reaction to that.

"Most people don't react to this one," Mary assured me. More saline, more Benadryl, then the carboplatin, and she was right. Uneventful. It was again six p.m. when we finished. I was exhausted and relieved to be done. What I was going through was sheer hell.

I looked at Mike and said, "I'm getting a frigging Quarter Pounder with cheese and large fries and a gigantic root beer."

He smiled lovingly at me. "Anything you want. I think you've earned it."

We eventually got home and I was happy that I knew more of what to expect. I was well prepared and heavily armed. With determination I started pounding back the water the minute I walked through the door, and I set several different alarms for pain relief—Claritin twice daily; Tylenol every four hours; Advil every six; hydromorphone every four to six hours, depending on whether I was awake; alarms for water, for electrolytes, steroids, sodium broths, and for checking my temperature.

Again I was in severe pain over the next several days, but because I was loaded up on a lot of drugs, I miraculously managed to stay out of emerg this time. I heavily credit Lara and Mike for this success. They kept a watchful eye on things. Lara stayed with me every day while Mike worked. In the evenings they took turns refilling my water, rubbing pain relief creams into my back and feet, and cooking amazing recovery meals. Again I was almost completely bedridden for the first ten days but not nearly as severely destroyed this time.

Social Media Post #8
April 25

Chemo round 2 update ♡

Hi peeps ☺ Soo nice to feel such support from all of you. A few people lately have been asking how I did with Round #2. (I was going to wait until I got through this week to really get a full understanding of how I reacted to it this round, but since people are asking, here I am! ♡) For starters, everybody that wished that the IV insertion would go smoothly this time, it did! They got it in

on the first try! I believe this is because the day before, I fully saturated my body with water, and those veins were waiting! However,
the chemo part did NOT go smoothly at all. I had an anaphylactic
reaction. It was no fun. I started seeing stars and trying not to pass
out. They had to give me adrenalin and Benadryl and steroids as
my breathing got laboured, and my mouth got very dry and my
tongue thick. It's amazing how quickly they reacted. That was with
only 25ml out of 175. After I got settled and they got an EKG of
my heart to make sure that the adrenalin was OK, they explained
that they can override the body's reaction with more Benadryl and
by starting the chemo IV drip very slowly. It was quite scary but,
miraculously, that is what they did. They managed to get the full
bag in me! The last two weeks I have been managing fairly well.
That still means I've been mostly bedridden, on hydromorphone
every four hours, but a lot less pain and a lot less nausea and up
until now no trips to emerg this time! Yay! I met with my oncologist
today and discussed my allergic reaction and she discussed all
of the different options. We are going ahead again this coming
Tuesday with round three of the same chemos. However, she is
going to give me steroids 12 hours before and 6 hours before and
then a slightly less amount of the chemo itself. That will be Round
#3. Then I will be halfway done my chemo! I will then have Round
#4 followed by 27 rounds of radiation and two more rounds of
chemo. We are getting there. I likely will not be able to respond to
all of you but would sure enjoy some hearts from everyone in the
comments to cheer me on. ♡

Love you all!

Sincerely, Egghead ☺

About day thirteen, Mike took Duey over to the family cottage for a
quiet walk, and I was in the kitchen with my sister. Lara could see I was
improving, and she got a twinkle in her eye. "Andrea," she said, enthusiastically, "I want to teach you how to do an ancient Shamanic practice for

energy-release work. It's quite powerful and I think it would be good for you, but I have to warn you, it's a little odd." She stood there, grinning. She was excited, happy, and feeling playful. I was a little unsure. I was worried; I know that face, I've known it my entire life. That face usually means I am on the receiving end of an impish practical joke. I reasoned that she knew how sick I was, so whatever she was about to do was likely not going to harm me.

"Uh, okay," I replied, hesitantly.

"Great!" She clapped her hands. "Okay. This practice is a movement form to help you release blocked energy, old beliefs, and traumas. It will help make room for healing. Stand up," she instructed.

I slowly pulled myself up to a standing position, my heart instantly pounding. "I don't have a lot of energy, Lara, just so you know."

"That's okay, I'll hold you if it comes to that. We will go slowly. Okay, watch what I do."

She spread her feet and slowly started moving her hips in large, slow circles. I started giggling. She looked weird.

"This is a really good movement; it gets energy flowing in each of your chakras," she said. "Try it!"

I stood there, caught off guard. *Oh gosh, I hate this stuff.* I felt awkward and self-conscious standing there in my ill-fitting, giant dress and bald head.

"Try it!" she said again. Knowing how keen she was, I slowly moved my hips in a small circle. I had to hang on to the edge of the table not to lose my balance. "Bigger." she instructed. I tried harder. "Make the biggest circles you can!" she called over the noise of wind suddenly blowing hard against the windows. I moved my hips around even more, yet I was stiff and careful as I continued to have pain from the hysterectomy, even after twelve weeks.

At this point I started feeling a little more comfortable. I could see she was serious about the benefits and was not at all laughing at me. I was still, however, waiting for a camera to secretly record me or something.

"Okay, great. That's it! Now, we are going to make a sound with the back of our throat. Make the lowest note you can make in a relaxed, gravelly voice. These deep guttural sounds represent unspoken words or thoughts that are not yet fully formed or consciously accessible. Just let your voice sit there." She opened her mouth wide, relaxed her throat, and slowly expelled a low, vibrating, foreign sound.

This, I knew how to do. As a music teacher, I had made similar sounds in vocal lessons, although not with the intent of Shamanic release work.

"AhhHHHhhhhHHHHhhhHHH." We stood there making this strange, eerie sound while swiveling our hips.

"Okay, good! That's good! Keep going!" she pushed.

I kept going.

"How are you doing? Are you feeling okay?"

"Yes."

"Good. Now we are going to bend over at the waist and ground our left foot and use it to pivot around with our right foot."

What? I stopped what I was doing and looked at her.

"Want me to show you?" She was so happy.

"Yes please." *Oh dear Lord what have I gotten myself into.*

"Okay!" she replied, smiling, and she confidently jumped right into it. I watched in fascination as she went from Anglo-Saxon white girl to some sort of ancient tribalist performing a primal ritual, right before my very eyes. She bent low at the hip, lowered her eyes to the floor. She dug her right foot down hard and pushed it, causing her to turn in circles.

"AhhaaaAHHHaaaaAHHHaaaaAAAAHHH." She was making low, animal sounds. Suddenly she stomped hard on the floor with her right foot, making the dishes rattle. "AhhaaaAHHHaaaaAHHHaaaaAAAAHHH," she sounded again, shaking her head back and forth in time with the stomping. I just stared at her, not knowing what to make of this demonstration.

I envisioned myself in a grassy field in Upper Canada somewhere, perhaps the Prairies, on ancient soil in a very different time. She continued on, loudly making primal sounds while spinning and shaking her head and stomping faster and faster. It was completely, unequivocally the most powerful and transformative thing I have ever witnessed. This went on for a full minute and I was now both mesmerized and completely stunned at the scene before me. This was not my sister as I had known her; this truly was another energy form, in another world. And then as abruptly as she had started, she finished, stood upright, and looked at me.

"Your turn!" she said, as if this wasn't the weirdest, funniest thing I had ever witnessed. It was especially shocking coming from her, my formerly quiet, somewhat shy, reserved sister.

I stood there, speechless and staring. I did not know what to make of this tribal dance, energy release work.

She waited, then realized something was wrong. "What?" she asked, trying to understand why I continued to just gape and not move.

The fact that she seemed so genuinely questioning of my reaction, as if I was the one who was unusual at this moment, made the scenario all the funnier. I tried my darndest to be respectful of her practice and teachings but could not contain my utter astonishment and amusement any longer. I cracked up laughing in true fits and giggles. I thought this was a joke now for sure.

"I told you it was a little odd, but honestly, it's so good for you. Just try it." she coaxed.

I struggled, not knowing what to say or even how to begin. "Lara, this is waaay out of my comfort zone, I don't even know how to start."

"Oh you have to do it, it feels amazing! It's just you and me here. I've wanted to show you this for days, but I knew Mike would think it weird and I didn't want to upset Duey."

She stood there nodding, like, *C'mon.* I took a deep breath and actually thought about it for a few seconds. *Nope.* "I don't think I can. I am not that open with my body to freely jump into such . . . such . . . reckless abandon. Like, I feel paralyzed to even start."

I felt really awkward. How does one give up control over their body to do this? It was so foreign. I was amazed to learn that I wasn't okay with potentially looking that foolish, even after a lifetime of being an entertainer. It was hard to understand and to accept.

Lara thought for a moment. "Just bend over, open your mouth, do the low voice thing, and use your foot to turn you. C'mon! Mike will be home soon and we will lose our chance."

I let out a deep sigh. She was pretty insistent and convincing. I bent over. I opened my mouth. I started to make the low growling throat noise. Carefully I put my foot down and turned a bit as I pushed.

"That's good! Get louder and stomp your foot, hard," she coached.

Suddenly, I felt like, *Screw it. I trust her, and there is no judgment. I'm doing this.* I gave it my all. I stomped my foot hard while pushing it into the floor, and it propelled me in a circle.

"Louder," she coached again, as I allowed my mouth to hang open and the sound to release.

"AhhaaaAHHHaaaaAHHHaaaaAAAAHHH" came out of me. Suddenly, all the anguish, anger, pain, fear, and emotional turmoil I had been faced with was washing around in my stomach and I had to get it out. "AhhaaaAHHHaaaaAHHHaaaaAAAAHHH," I intoned again, this time with more strength and power. My eyes started watering. I stomped and spun. "AhhaaaAHHHaaa—ack!" The sound suddenly stuck in my throat and I gagged. Hard. I felt like I was going to throw up. Drool came out of my mouth in a big long string as tears fell from my eyes.

"Keep going! You are clearing negative energy!" Lara called to me.

Around and around I circled and stomped, flashbacks of Nurse Evil, my cancer news, the pain, the chemo, all of it. "AhhaaaAHHHaaa—ack!" I tried again, and gagged even harder. I had to stop. Winded and breathless, I stood upright, swaying from side to side, panting and wiping my mouth with my sleeve. Shyly, I looked at Lara.

"Andrea! That was incredible. How do you feel?"

I thought for a moment. I felt lighter. Happy, actually. Yes. "I feel happy!" In fact, I couldn't believe how good I felt.

"Andrea, I see energy in the form of colours. I saw dark grey strands coming off of your body and out of your mouth. When you gagged, you released deep, stuck energy that was trapped in your body! You have done very well with this. You have experienced profound, powerful healing." Lara looked incredibly pleased.

"Really?" I asked. I wanted so desperately to understand and to believe it was helpful. At a minimum it was a lesson in trust, to allow myself to participate in something I felt very uncomfortable doing.

"Yes! It was quite remarkable!" Lara confirmed.

This debriefing went on for a minute or so longer and then Mike and Duey came through the doors, narrowly missing my "ancient, shamanic, tribal-release." I was startled by their arrival. Mike saw the two of us standing there breathless and smiling.

"'Sup?" Mike asked, looking back and forth between the two of us.

We stood there, energized and laughing. I briefly tried to describe what we were doing while Lara reassured him that she took her time, slowly and carefully assessing me all the way, making sure I was well hydrated and not dizzy or getting light-headed. Mike pushed past us and opened the fridge. I could tell he was not really into this stuff, but I already knew that.

Hours later we were sitting around the table snacking while Mike barbecued. Music played and I felt energized. I longed for a wild night of dancing and booze. "I really wish I could have some wine," I announced as I watched Lara and Mike raising their glass. It made me recall happier days gone by. I missed the taste and the mellow, relaxed feeling I'd get halfway through glass number two. I had tried wine once while on chemo a few weeks back and it had tasted awful to me. This was exceedingly weird because, I LOVE wine.

"Have one of your chocolates," Mike suggested.

"Nah," I replied.

We had a friend who had a "specialty" chocolate business. She was a master crafter and could make any flavour or strain of party chocolate you wanted. She crafted one for me that helped me sleep and took my mind off chemo and my current misery. "The best thing you'll need during your treatments," she had promised. They *were* delicious and they did help me sleep. But I wanted something to make me feel upbeat and giggly, and typically that was wine. In the past prior to chemo, I'd discovered anything other than alcohol didn't agree with my system, and I dutifully steered clear.

"Try half of one and see if you feel relaxed. If not, don't bother with the other half." Mike got up and went to the fridge where I stored them.

"What is this chocolate you're talking about?" Lara asked.

I explained it to her. I had purchased twenty-five of them months ago and still had about ten left. "Want one?" I asked.

"Are they strong?"

"No, they are specifically used as a mellow sleep aid. There is no THC at all."

She thought for a moment, and I added, "They are really yummy—high quality chocolate with sea salt and caramel."

"Okay." Lara shrugged. We'd been craving sweets too. We each ate a half.

Dinner was assembled and eaten, and thirty minutes later we sat at the table telling very funny stories and laughing really hard. I wasn't sure if it was the stories or the chocolates that made us laugh that hard, and I reminded myself that the chocolates were not very strong, therefore assumed it was just the true gladness of sisters reminiscing. Lara's face reflected what I felt too—utter joy and sheer bliss. I felt really good. I had had these chocolates before and I hadn't felt THAT happy. I mean, we had perma-smiles on our faces.

I started to question the chocolates when the phone rang and I sort of mildly panicked, not sure if I should answer. It was an odd feeling.

"Lara! Mom's calling. She wants to FaceTime." I looked at my sister, wondering what to do. She looked a little uncertain too. I opened my camera and checked out my smiling face. I rationalized I was genuinely just immensely happy and decided to answer.

"Hello, Mama." I sang, seeing her face smiling at me. Mom wanted to know what we were up to and how I was feeling. We talked for a bit and then Mike went out to scrape the BBQ and turn it off.

He came back in and said, "You're not gonna wanna miss this sunset. Come check it out!" Lara hopped up immediately, and I slowly followed behind. I told Mom I was going to put the phone down for a brief moment so I could stand for a picture with the sunset behind me, and then Lara, Mike, and I got completely caught up in the mesmerizing beauty of it all.

"Wow," Lara said, blown away by the beautiful, spiritual scene.

"Nice, eh?" Mike replied.

"Oh my gosh, that is just glorious!" I exclaimed. We just stood there, happily staring at the giant, glowing orb and pink clouds so artistically dispersed in a blue sky. We took a few more photos and just stood there, breathing in the ocean air, listening to the crashing surf and watching the sun drop low on the horizon. I have no idea how many minutes passed, but at a minimum I would guess at least five.

All of a sudden we heard Mom's voice behind us. "Well this is fun." she groaned, making us all jump.

Startled and confused, Lara and I quickly looked at each other. "Wait, where's Mom?" Lara asked. We had forgotten Mom! She was still waiting on FaceTime, placed on the table and stuck staring up at the roof.

This struck us both as so terribly funny, we went into whoops and hollers and had tears streaming down our faces. Chemo and my hysterectomy had damaged my bladder control, so I went racing into the bathroom screeching, "I'm going to pee! Move it! I'm going to PEE!" I hobbled with my knees pressed together and my hand wrapped around my front trying not to leak. Lara and Mike could not stop laughing. Ultimately, Mike took the phone from Lara and kept talking to Mom as Lara continued robustly laughing in the living room.

In the bathroom by myself, I too was laughing. Each time I settled down I could hear Lara still laughing in the living room by herself and it got me started all over again. I came out and she hurried over to me. "Andrea," she whispered so Mom wouldn't overhear, "did you know she was still on the phone? Did you forget about her? Her voice came out of nowhere and totally startled me!" This cracked me up even more. I couldn't tell if she was joking or serious. She was just so silly, and this got me going all over again.

We ended the call with Mom, and our relaxed, happy state lasted several more hours into the night as we laid on the couches with our feet up. We talked and talked. It was one of the happiest moments in my cancer journey and a really special one with my sister. We solved the world's problems that evening, and then some.

The next morning, I explained that the chocolates had never had that effect on me before. We credited the energy clearing we had done in the afternoon, which made us highly receptive to the chocolates.

"Andrea, your birthday is coming up in a few days. I'd like to make your favourite cake for you." I was again surprised at all of her loving efforts.

I thought for a moment. I could not recall the last time someone had made a cake for me, and I was very touched. Carrot cake was my favourite. "I have a carrot cake recipe that everyone loves," I told Lara. "It is a ton of work. I make it for Mike and our friends on their birthdays, and they all love it. I have never had anyone make it for me. I wouldn't ask you to do it, as it is so much work. Could you maybe *buy* me a carrot cake?"

"Andrea, I will make it for you. You give me the recipe. I'm not getting you a store-bought cake. You are worth a thousand homemade carrot cakes on your birthday. You deserve it."

This brought tears to my eyes as I again struggled with my self-worth.

28

CHEMO ROUND #3 AND THE POTASSIUM HORROR

If you asked me if I was nervous about getting chemo round #3 after my very upsetting anaphylactic reaction to #2, I would tell you that quite honestly, I feared for my life. Knowing how quickly and violently I had reacted to the infusion only three short weeks ago made me extremely hesitant to go back.

A few days before this next round, my dear friend Sue had come to visit and had given me a lovely gift basket that included, of all things, two rubber, gel-infused frogs. Similar to stress balls, they were intended for me to squeeze during the next chemo while they were getting things set up for the unbearably stressful IV.

We had to trust the capabilities of the staff and of the medicine required. I had done my due diligence, setting alarms and taking steroids twelve and six hours before. Physically, I was as ready as I could be, but mentally—well, that was an entirely different story. I'll admit it; I was really struggling.

The drive in that morning was again beyond tense as I was just so completely, emotionally distressed about my current state of affairs. I was starting to feel immensely tired of the entire procedure.

Social Media Post #9

May 2

Heading in to the VG. Round #3. I had some tears last night.
Feeling a bit of dread mentally about the long road ahead and just
feeling a bit like a pin cushion with the constant blood work and
IVs every few weeks. People, your comments truly lift my spirits.
Like I said in an earlier post, I can't always reply because I sleep
so much now but wanted to express my sincere gratitude today
and every day for having you all with me on this journey. I feel
truly blessed.

Once again, I had to really focus, coaxing my body not to pass out as I
was, for another entire miserable hour, painfully poked five times. Needles
were going in and bursting, digging, and entirely missing veins, with three
different nurses making attempts. As awful as it was, it still ended up being
quite a colourful morning.

I survived the third chemo infusion and to my surprise did not have
a dangerous reaction during my time there. I was heavily sedated with
Benadryl and some steroids that were quite powerful, to override any potential reactions, big or small. I was to continue taking the steroids for several
more days while home, in order to avoid any further reactivity.

Social Media Post #10

May 2

Dear Friends,

Thank you for your encouraging words to me early this morning as I braved yet another round of chemo. There was a little bit
of levity at the chemo center today. I prepared for my IV as intently
as I could. Yesterday, I committed and focused on the much
needed task of proper hydration. I drank 100 oz. of water. I medi-
tated. I envisioned a smooth needle insertion by the nurse, and I

asked my body to allow the needle on the first attempt. I practiced slow, deep, controlled breaths. They know as a redhead, my veins are trouble. Small, deep, rolling veins and thick skin makes for a novice needler's nightmare. I had new-to-me girl and we prepared. I calmly explained my veins, and even though my left arm is worse, they said protocol dictates they try alternate arms each chemo round in order to protect veins. So we soaked my left arm for five minutes in a tub of hot water. Then out came the oven-warmed flannel towels. Then came the tight, rubber bands, vein searching, and poking. Lots of "hmms," lots of looking.

After two painful, failed attempts, the nurse explained again that "We only get two attempts and then we must fetch a colleague to try." By this point I was getting anxious, so I pulled out my stress ball. It calms me and also as I squeeze, it helps the veins get bigger. So I'm squeezing the $h!t out of my stress ball, (which today was one of the purple gel frogs from a dear friend,) except the nurse didn't know I had it and couldn't see it in my tightly closed fist as the large, flannel arm wrap was hiding it. All of the sudden we both heard a loud "POP!" A pile of blue gel shot straight out from the end of the blanket. It quickly went all over her Lulu pants and all over the floor!! ☺ She was shocked and jumped as the gel blopped everywhere, and I too was quite surprised. Of course the first thing that popped into my mind is a pregnancy joke. "Oh my gosh, my water broke!" I decried loudly with a horrified, panicked face. The nurse looked completely confused and I began laughing loud, hysterical belly laughs at my own joke. Feeling a little awkward now, I pulled the frog out from under the blanket and relieved it from my clenched fist as more blue gel spilled out on me. It was a total mess. Sheepishly I explained that the frog was used as my stress ball. She looked at me in concern and awe and then asked, "How hard were you squeezing your frog?" ☺ A loud scene ensued as other chemo patients watched this messy moment unfold. Wet, messy, glopping piles of bright

blue gel were everywhere, and a dead, deflated rubber frog lay
lifeless on the floor. Moral of the story, dollar-store frogs are NOT
for chemo patients. Oh, and the IV attempts today? FIVE; three
different nurses, one hour of effort.

I enjoyed reading the responses from that post on my way home, as the chemo slowly began to take hold. Now, you may recall Dr. Scott was very emphatic that if I were to develop a fever of over 100.4 I was to go directly to emerg. I had done this back in Round #1. I had fevers in Round #2, but I figured out that if I was at all dehydrated, my body was not able to effectively clear the dying mass of cells that the chemo was killing. My body then elevated my temp to kill those dead cells and toxins as an invader. I had watched my body fluctuate and hover back and forth numerous times, and it seemed my temp would lower a bit after an influx of water. I figured I was not in any danger to stay home from emerg even though time and time again I was plagued with fevers. Emerg was miserable and dreadfully slow, and I was more comfortable isolating and monitoring. However, this particular round of chemo hit me exceedingly hard.

Much like chemo Round #1, I was completely bedridden and in severe pain. It was at least more manageable than the first round, but only marginally so. Lara had flown back to California and was not around to help with my care while Mike worked. At about day six, I was not only in a weakened state from the chemo, but also having much more dangerous heart issues. Just from the effort of rolling over in bed, my heart rate would soar to 180. It felt dreadful. I could not get out of bed without fainting, and I struggled to stay awake and conscious. I decided with very little convincing this time that I indeed needed to make another trip to emerg.

Mike drove me in and I was happy to observe that this time, I was with a nurse and getting blood drawn within forty-five minutes of our arrival. Dr. Scott had been appalled when we told her during my checkup what had happened at Emergency after Round #1. She promised she would make a phone call and review with the staff what the protocol was and the importance of it, and I was very happy to see things had improved. Within an hour of arriving I now had my own room safely away from all others in emerg. I could lie down in the bed with a flannel sheet and have protection from any potential COVID exposure or other bug out in the main area.

As usual, the blood work did not go well, and I was told I would need yet another IV for yet another CT scan to check for any potential clots. At this point, I continued to have abdominal pain.

I had the tests and we waited several more hours for results. They discovered that my neutrophils were dangerously low, at zero. If I was exposed to any type of bacterial or viral infection at all, my body would be extremely challenged to fight it off. The neutrophil's job is to defend against the invader. Zero neutrophils meant no defender. They also discovered that my potassium was extremely low, which is what was making my heart rate skyrocket dangerously high. It was well into the evening when a nurse came in to get me set up with a potassium IV.

She was covered in tattoos, which left me quite uneasy; the largest tattoo was a full black python wrapped around her entire forearm with enormous, razor-sharp fangs. I couldn't stop looking at it. I have a phobia of snakes and was trying to adjust my eyes in the dimly lit room to make sure this wicked thing was indeed only a tattoo. The snake looked all too real, with fangs all too ready to sink into my arm.

"Okay, Andrea, I was sent to give you a potassium infusion," the nurse stated. I saw a small bag filled with white, cloudy liquid. "Have you ever had one before?" she asked, talking quickly, rushing. Emergency was a busy place and the hospital was understaffed.

"No," I mumbled, I was in rough shape and very tired.

"Okay, well . . . some people can't tolerate them, so you just let me know if it's bothersome, okay?"

Can't tolerate them. How odd. Does it cause an allergy? I guess all I can do is wait and see.

"Okay," I mumbled again. She attached the potassium bag to the IV pole and inserted the drip tube to the bottom of the bag, adjusting it as there were a few air bubbles.

Once it started dripping, she looked at me. "All good?" she asked.

"All good," I replied as the first few drops entered my arm. She promptly left.

Literally two seconds after she closed the door, my arm felt like it was on fire. *Oh no, this is burning. Ow. Holy crap. OW! Oh my God . . .*

I sat up, quickly going from almost asleep to intense pain. My adrenalin surged into a fight or flight reaction. "Hello!" I yelled, and could only manage to wait two seconds before I started sobbing. I began to panic. I looked at my arm to see if it was going to explode right in front of me. My heart started to race even faster as the pain became extreme. "Hello! Help me! Quick! This is burning me BADLY!" I was terrified at how immediate the pain was. I waited, writhing in pain and panicking. No one came.

The pain became even more intense than extreme. It was *destroying* me. I started panting and breathing deep, concentrated breaths, trying to control the pain but to no avail. I can't imagine what my heart rate was at this point, and I am sure my blood pressure was well up in the "stroke zone." My head jerked to the door and my eyes searched the window above; the nurses' station was just on the other side. Still no response. Desperate, I looked for a way to pull the IV out of my arm. It was firmly taped down. I scrambled to sit completely upright to find a button on the machine to stop the IV drip, all the while whimpering and writhing. Covered in sweat, I began vocalizing this bizarre "Hehhh-hehhh-hehhh-hehhh" sound as I couldn't stand the intense potassium destroying the veins in my arm even a second longer.

I reached the frantic level as I looked for a hospital button to ring the nurse and then saw that she had not bothered to fasten one in a reachable spot. I checked my arm again to make sure it was not about to explode and then desperately lunged to the side of the bed trying to reach the intercom pull cord with my fingertips. I just barely caught the red line for it. Unbelievably, it escaped my fingers. "C'mon, Andrea!" I yelled in sheer frustration and panic as I knew no one could save me. "Grab it," I ordered myself, my teeth clenched. I stretched again and felt my muscles tighten and ache in my back as I reached desperately for that cord. I made contact and it fell into my palm. I wrapped my fingers around it and yanked on it as hard as I could. "Hehhh-hehhh-hehhh-hehhh," I puffed and squirmed and panted and sweated, waiting desperately for a voice to answer.

"Yes?" a casual voice asked on the intercom. "Please come quickly! This IV is burning me badly!" I begged. I was now breathing so deeply I saw stars. My fingertips started to go numb. "Hurry!" I yelled. I looked at my arm in a crazy-eyed psychosis as I envisioned bright red veins filling up, expanding puffily under my skin, bursting wide open, and spraying bright red blood everywhere. It felt so horribly painful, that I kept checking my arm to see that it wasn't actually splitting into a tearing, burst-open, painful mess.

Finally, the nurse walked in and saw me twisting and turning and yelling and panting. "Oh dear!" she exclaimed, and ran the last few steps, hurriedly pressing the black button on the side of the machine. The liquid stopped. I laid there, still deeply panting, "hehhh-hehhh-hehhh-hehhh" as I struggled not to pass out or have a heart attack. The potassium drip ceased, but it took a full minute longer of heavy panting and squirming for the intense pain to ease and for my heart rate to stop wildly beating out of my heaving chest. I was shaking violently. I tried hard to control my breathing. Lips pursed, I heard the sounds coming from me but didn't understand them. My body was doing this all on its own, trying to restore itself. "Whooooo-heh-whooooo-heh-whooooo"—uneven, deep breaths, in and out. The nurse watched me for a moment and then said, "I guess you can't tolerate it, huh." I barely heard her over my deep breaths and near-blacking out.

Now people, I will firmly insist that you memorize my PSA: some people cannot tolerate potassium infusions. Please, re-read that and take it as a lesson. Know it. I had no idea that this was a thing. But let me tell you, nothing in all of my past life—the pain of the hysterectomy, the pain of the days following, the pain of delivering one of my daughters without an epidural, the pain of delivering the seven-pound clay baby, the horrible uterine biopsy, a dreaded laparoscopy, colonoscopies, the horrific chemo pain . . . *none* of these extremely painful moments in my life compared remotely to the indescribable, tortuous pain of this incident.

indescribable: too unusual, too intense, too extreme or indefinite to be adequately described. Beyond description.

torturous: involving excruciating pain or severe suffering. Agonizing. Harrowing.

pain: a localized or generalized unpleasant bodily sensation or complexity of sensations that causes mild to severe physical and emotional distress marked by acute shooting pains.

Now, I have had plenty of IVs. And I do mean *plenty*, many more than the average person, I would say. And some of them have stung a great deal. Pushing liquid chemicals through teeny-tiny, chemo-burned, shrunken veins is not easy to handle, but I have managed to power through. There have been times the IV hurt so much it caused me to clench my teeth and my toes, it took my breath away; and even brought me to tears.

The potassium IV infusion was quite honestly the closest thing I would compare to actual physical torture. It was an entirely new level of pain, *indescribable and tortuous*. I was so shocked by how exceptionally painful my episode was, I did some research in the days following to understand why it was so horrific. It has since been determined that the potassium level was too concentrated, it was infused too quickly, I did not receive a numbing agent, and my veins were already too burned and too small from the chemo to be remotely receptive of the potassium.

When I was finally able to speak, I cried out in total disbelief. "Oh my God! That was horrible! People can actually get that *in*?" I was incredulous. I vowed this was never going to happen to me again. It was indescribably horrific.

"Yeah, I think it's sort of like how some people get stinky pee when they eat asparagus, and some don't." She smiled at me, completely oblivious to my inordinate amount of pain. "Okay. We are going to try this again, but slower. We can usually get it in slower."

My adrenalin soared and I felt quite angry all of a sudden. Enough was enough. "No! Absolutely not! I refuse." I looked at her fiercely. There was no way. No. Way. I was still panting and my heart still racing.

She shrugged. "Okay," was all she said. She left the room.

Another nurse came in. She smiled at me, a new tactic. "Andrea, we need to try to give you this medicine. Your heart is in a dangerous situation. You need to get the potassium in you."

"No," I said firmly, crossing my arms.

"We can do it slower. It won't be nearly as bad."

"No!" I said louder, more firmly. I was not going to do this at all.

"Okay, I'll see about getting you some potassium tablets." She said and started to walk out.

What the actual hell. "Wait. There are *tablets* for this?" I was yelling now. "Why would anyone agree to a drip when there are tablets?" I was completely mystified why anyone would choose this liquid torture. It was worse than getting your fingernails pulled out—of that I am certain.

"Because it is more accurate and faster than the pill form," she answered. "The pill only comes in one dosage, but the liquid can be in millilitres."

"Please go get me the pills," I groaned, collapsing back on the bed in tears.

A while later Sue came in to visit me. I tried to explain the pain to her. I am not sure anyone will ever know the pain of this experience, unless they pour a vat of acid in their eye, light themselves on fire with gasoline, and then chop off all of their toes one at a time while pouring apple cider vinegar on the raw, exposed tips. That might give a sense of the immense pain. It was, worse than *anything*.

The nurse reappeared. "Andrea, we are going to admit you. The doctor feels you are too unwell to be home right now."

Oh for the love of God, no. "Really? Is that necessary?" I politely asked, thinking that would change their minds.

"Your numbers are too troublesome," she explained, looking somewhat relieved she was off the hook. And, off we went, with more paramedics and another ambulance.

By then it was two in the morning and I had been transported to the cancer floor of the Victoria General Hospital. The paramedics slid a hard white plastic surfboard-type thing under me on my cot and then lifted me up and placed me down on the hospital bed. They pulled out the surfboard and wrapped me in blankets. They were really kind. "Best of luck with everything!" they called over their shoulders as they left. I looked around. *I have a room all to myself.* No dirty bathrooms, no other interruptions with different visitors and food drop-offs. *This is a nice surprise!*

A nurse came in and said, "Did you get your potassium yet?" and I realized I hadn't gotten the pills.

"No, not yet," I replied politely. She left quietly and came back in. She began hooking up my IV again as it had been taken apart at the other hospital and the entry site carefully wrapped.

I watched her like a hawk. All of a sudden she took a white liquid bag out of her pocket. "Is that an IV bag of potassium?" I asked nervously, trying to sit up. My heart raced again from the stress and the physical effort of getting upright.

"Yes, it is," she said, perhaps wondering how I knew.

"I'm not having that," I said firmly. *Gosh, that sounds rude.*

"No?" She was kind, I could tell, but she was determined to do her job.

"They said I could have pills."

She sighed a wee bit. "The doctor here says we need the liquid."

I felt my lips trembling. I politely but firmly explained what had happened only a short while ago. She politely and firmly explained she needed to follow the doctor's orders. We carefully danced the "dance of negotiation" for a good five minutes. She was working on me, saying, "I will do it much, much slower, it will not be nearly as bad."

Surprisingly, she managed to win me over. I foolishly reasoned that since my body overrode the anaphylactic response only just five days ago with the chemo because *it* was slower, maybe, perhaps, I could manage to get this stuff in.

"Okay, I will try, but please don't go far in case I suddenly need you."

She smiled reassuringly at me and I trusted her. Moments later she started it up, assured me again that it would be fine on a slower speed, and left. And seconds later, the same horror show began, except this time, with my veins being already highly sensitive and irritated, the pain was even more severe. When you experience torture, the body reacts in extremely uncontrollable ways. I came very close to screaming, and even though I knew there were people dying on this floor and it was the middle of the night, I almost lost that last ounce of control. My body was on the verge of a total breakdown. With every ounce of strength I had left, I tried my hardest to tolerate the slower potassium drip, and that effort lasted all of three seconds.

"Help me!" I bellowed so loudly I swear people on the other side of the city heard me. The nurse came running back in. She pushed the button and stopped the machine.

"I will go call the doctor," she said breathlessly, and raced out. I laid there, panting and grabbing my arm. I looked at my watch to check my heart rate: 196 bpms. I cried and panted and laid there covered in sweat for a good three minutes before my heart rate returned to 130, a more normal rate for me. I was beside myself. I could not take any more.

The nurse returned with a yellow banana full of dark brown spots. It stunk the worst ripe banana smell I have ever smelled. "Can you try to eat this?" she smiled gently at me. I like my bananas just a minute past green, like, under ripe. This was the entire other side of ripe.

"Is this in place of the drip?" I asked. I would eat it as a trade.

"No, it is not."

I peeled it. I slowly put my teeth around it and took one careful, slow bite. Just as my teeth bit into the banana, I gagged a violent, forceful gag, and the food hadn't even gotten in my mouth. "I can't, I'm sorry."

I will never forget the next moment as long as I live. She looked very guilty and apologetic by what she was about to do. What she did, was unquestionably the worst moment in all of my entire life. She fidgeted with numbers on the machine, pressed the black button to turn the IV back on, and then quickly walked out of the room. I knew she had again lowered the speed in a last-ditch effort to get the very much needed potassium in me. She was told by the doctor to get it done.

In horror, I watched as the potassium dripped very slowly down the IV line. I knew it would only be a matter of seconds before the severe burning in my veins would start again for an unthinkable third time. This beautiful, kind, patient nurse was now my torturer. And then, there it was. This nightmare of searing, burning, stinging, unfathomable pain in my veins, travelling up my arm, and burning the nerves.

"Help me now, please! Turn this off!" I screamed as loud as I could muster. "Aaahhh!" And then realizing that I had seen the other hospital nurse press a big black button, I took a risk and lunged for the machine and managed to turn it off. I fell back into bed, panting, crying, yelling, "Give me the damn pills! Why won't you just listen to me?" I felt horrible that I could not get the message across without turning into a writhing, screaming lunatic, covered in sweat.

The nurse came in again, her face filled with pity and guilt. "Okay, Andrea. I will call the doctor again and get you the pills. You stay tight."

I laid there, delusional, breathless, and terrified. Panting deeply, crying, alone. I truly expected my heart to give up and go into some crazy arrhythmia at any moment and that I would die in the next few minutes. It was a miserable, lonely experience, and I told myself that I loved myself very much and that I was going to be okay, even if I *did* die.

The nurse came back in after a few moments and handed me a small paper cup with two very large pills. I took them hastily. Without a word, she left, and I fell deeply asleep until the morning, when, you guessed it, I was awakened for more needles and more blood work.

The day was pretty uneventful. A few hours into the morning, one of the nurses came in at the end of her shift as my IV machine had been beeping. (When the IV machines beep, the nurses need to check them to understand what caused the alarm to go off. Sometimes it's just a signal that a fluid bag is done, but other times it signals a problem with the line.) She tapped the side of the machine. It beeped some more. She opened up a flap and pulled the line out and snapped it three times to break up the bubbles. She put it back inside the flap part and the beeping continued.

"I don't really know what's wrong with this thing, so I'm just going to get you a whole new line; sometimes that's what it needs." She left quickly and came back with a lengthy amount of tubing and changed it.

I think perhaps she forgot to press "forward" on the line as now she chatted away and I listened to her for a minute before feeling pain in my arm at my IV site. Exhausted, still heavily stressed and needing to just decompress, I could not believe my eyes. More horror as I saw my blood now travelling out of my arm and back up the clear line. About twelve inches of bright red blood had been sucked back up the tube. Now, maybe to an experienced nurse or doctor, this is nothing, but to me? This was absolutely dreadful.

"Uh, what's happening here?" I asked, looking at the blood and trying not to lose my cool.

"Oh, whoops!" she said and pressed another button.

I watched my blood go back down the tube and then *back in* my arm. It was very upsetting. She continued talking about her dog as if that moment was an everyday, run-of-the-mill thing. For me, it was not, and it added just one more layer of deep worry and trauma to my already heavily stacked list.

I was admitted for three long days and was replenished with sodium, potassium, calcium, magnesium, fluids, and lots of pain meds. When I was finally feeling physically better, I was greatly relieved to be released. I was booked in for another consult with oncology to discuss chemo Round #4, scheduled for more blood work before the next round, and was pretty much ready to jump off a bridge.

29
CHEMO ROUND #4

The chemo consult for Round #4 was the usual. In addition to the checkup, I told Dr. Scott that I had numbing in my fingers and toes and was concerned by this, as I am a guitar teacher and wasn't sure how badly this was going to affect my ability to play. It was quite troubling. Neuropathy is a common complication with chemo. Unfortunately, I was too weak to play my guitar to even assess how bad it was. We discussed the plan of using less chemo at a lower dose for the next round to see if this would alleviate the numbness, the severe bone pain, and the effects on my neutrophils and potassium levels. Mentally, I pushed through and agreed to more chemo, all the while feeling completely miserable and totally anxious. I was losing my desire to fight through it all, hating my life more and more every minute.

Following the chemo meeting was the radiation appointment. With my head still spinning from the decision to carry on with the chemo, I headed around the corner to the radiation centre and numbly sat through another meeting, more plans, more decisions, and more information, doing my best to learn all about the upcoming radiation. While there I had to drink 500 ml of water followed by a scan and tattoos. This scan was in preparation for the actual set-up and positioning of the radiation machines. I met with the staff and perked up when I learned today's scan did not involve dye or IVs. They were most impressed with my ability to chug the water back quite quickly (a throwback perhaps to my university days?) and I was brought to the radiation room for the marking procedures. A very friendly radiation technician (rad tech) greeted me and was an absolute breath of fresh air as I got up on the table. She explained that I was there to get a tattoo to mark the spots needed for consistent positioning with each session of the radiation.

"Have you ever had a tattoo before?" the rad tech asked.

Once before, years ago, I'd had the experience of being tattooed with my sister and recalled the day quite vividly . . .

We were roughly twenty-three and twenty-two, driving to New Brunswick for old time's sake, on our way to surprise our now *very* senior Nana. On the drive there, we decided to take a break and find some lunch. We stopped at a small eatery about two hours from our destination and got talking to the locals. When we told them we were from out of town, they told us to make sure we stopped at the "World Famous Tattoo Parlour" just up the street. Now, before that day, Lara and I had never even considered tattoos, but it was the beginning of the next generation's rage of shoulder tattoos, ankle tattoos and on occasion maybe even one's lower back. We laughed at the thought of getting one and joked about how horrified our mother would be had we chosen to do so. Over lunch, this idea turned into a real topic of conversation, and we decided just for kicks to go to the parlour for some investigating.

Nervously we entered into an "adults-only" shop and three men greeted us warmly at the door. The place stank of cigarettes and much worse, but we were raised to be polite and stayed long enough for them to discover we were from out of town, never had a tattoo and were mildly curious. Fast forward a few moments later and they presented us with two giant three-ringed binders that covered every tattoo from bumble bees to large breasted biker-chicks, from Jesus wearing a halo to skulls and confederate flags. We were a little overwhelmed and politely declined any artwork.

"Well," one of the burlier men asked, "what kinda things are you girls into?"

We shrugged. "I play trombone . . ." I heard my voice trail off. I certainly wasn't going to get a *trombone* put anywhere on my body.

"I like frogs." Lara chirped in.

"We got frogs in here somewhere . . ." the man proclaimed, drawing a long haul off his cigarette. "Hang on just a sec." He expertly thumbed through a binder and located a small, leaping frog, the size of a quarter.

"75 bucks for that guy." He said. "Any color you want."

This intrigued Lara. "Do you have purple?" she asked shyly.

"Sure do!" he replied.

Lara looked at me, daring. I looked back at her. "Do you want a frog?" she asked, nervously hopeful. I didn't like frogs at all. I reminded her that when we were kids at the cottage she used to fetch them in a bucket at the frog pond and terrify me with them.

"Uh . . . I don't really have a reason to get a frog . . ." I said, disappointed. Lara wanted us to find something we both liked, something the same . . . a special "sister connection."

"Do ya speak any French?" the guy asked again, blowing smoke rings just past my face. "A little bit." I replied and then Lara got that familiar gleam in her eye. "Her boyfriend is French!" she disclosed, now looking so very happy.

"Ah! Well, there ya go! Your frog can be for that. You know, (another long drag on the cigarette) the nick name for the French is . . . "The Frog." What color do you want?"

I was quite taken aback. This was all moving waaay too fast. "I-I'm not really sure I want a tattoo today, thank you." I half stammered.

"Tell ya what, I'll do them both for 125 bucks. That's a real' good deal."

Lara looked at me. We had no idea if it was actually a "real' good deal" at the time, but looking back now, I know that that price was quite exorbitant and they likely laughed us all the way to the bank.

"Andrea, let's go get a drink and discuss this. I think I might do it!" I was amazed at how badly my sister wanted that purple frog. "Where will you put it?" I asked, trying to imagine a purple blob somewhere on my own body.

"Maybe on my hip?" she thought for a moment. "Yes, then no one will see it if I don't want them to see." Hmm, it *sounded* reasonable enough.

I decided I would think about it. We told the men we would be back after we went to get some cash at a local bank, and on our way we ended up finding a pool hall. We had a few drinks and played a few messy rounds of pool. I was starting to come around to the tattoo idea, but didn't like the color purple with my bright red hair. "Get green" Lara suggested, "it'll look good with your skin tone and your big green eyes." We downed two more drinks and nervously walked back to the tattoo parlour. The men were quite pleased to see us again. "Who's up first?" Smoke ring guy asked. "She is" we both said, pointing to the other, half panicky. "Tell ya what, flip a coin." We did, and . . . sure enough, I "won" the chance to go first.

I pulled my jeans down just enough to show my hip and awkwardly laid there with this stranger's hands on me. The "artist" quickly began and I instantly felt a buzzy, painful, hot stinging on my skin. I knew if I squirmed or winced Lara might change her mind and I would never live it down if Mom found out that I got a tattoo. *Would Lara explain that she had chickened out? Or would she act like I was brazenly flying solo with this new trend?* I clenched my teeth and really focused on putting my mind elsewhere. "Yer doin' good, dear. Almost done." Mr. Smokey-smoke said.

"Oh my gosh Andrea, doesn't that hurt?" Lara asked, amazed.

Yes. It hurt quite a bit actually, but I lied. I looked her square in the eye.

"No, it tickles actually! It's not bad at all."

"Ok . . ." she replied, still unsure.

A few more minutes and I was finished; my delicate, fair skin already turning quite red and beginning to swell. "Yer up!" a tall, skinny guy nodded to Lara, as I excused myself to pay. I came back to see her in the chair with a scrunched up face, glaring at me. She had one leg bent at a funny angle all the way into her chest, her toes tightly clenched; her sandal looked like it was going to bend in two.

"Oh my God, Andrea! This KILLS." She looked annoyed and amazed that I hadn't flinched.

"Best. Joke. EVER!" I whispered as I smiled down at her; so happy I had finally managed to trick her.

Clearly she would *not* have followed through had I shown her how much it had stung. She looked like she was going to kill me but shortly after, it was all finished. The frogs actually looked really cute. We went on to our Nana's house and told her what we'd done. "Don't tell your Mother, whatever you do." Nana said, looking a little concerned. In those days, tattoos were for bikers and Navy guys and not much more. We promised we wouldn't tell our Mother, and she didn't actually find out for several more years. Perhaps it was when I was giving birth to my first born . . . Mom was in the delivery room with me for that.

"Have you ever had a tattoo before?" I heard the kind voice ask again. I quickly opened my eyes. The rad tech was looking over me.

"Oh yes!" I replied, showing her my small frog tattoo and another equally small but very special one.

"Oh, that's great. So this won't bother you one bit!" She got out her laser and measured something on my hips.

"Is my frog in the way?" I asked, worried.

"No, he's fine." She said smiling. "He's really sweet!"

And "ZAP!" just like that, she stung me with her gun.

"Ouch!" I cried, surprised to feel such pain.

"Whoops! Sorry, I might have poked a little deeper than I meant to." She zapped another dot tattoo on my pelvic bone and a third on my other hip. It was all fine after a few minutes.

"Those are the permanent markers for your radiation."

Cool, I thought. *Those dots, paired with my five angry looking scars from the hysterectomy, look just so attractive.*

The following scan ended up being a bit complicated with a lot of ups and downs and a few more measurements.

"All done!" she announced triumphantly.

I hurriedly got up and out as I was so very tired of all the poking and just plain being in a hospital.

"See you in about a week and a half." She called as I walked out.

Social Media Post #11

May 19

Hello friends,

Another chemo consult today before next Tuesday (round #4).

That meeting was then followed by my radiation appointments

to line up five weeks of daily radiation. (That involved having CT scans and little, tiny tattoos on my hips and pelvic area to set things up.) They told me to keep my underwear on when I was putting my hospital gown on. When I got into the CT room the tech said, "Bring your underwear down to your knees." This ended up being up-down-up-down-up-down as I had to interrupt the process to get more water to fill my bladder and then at one point we had to empty the bladder, as it was too full, so a lot of up and down with the underwear.

When we were all finished the scan and the little tattoos, the rad tech smiled and asked, "Well, how was that?" Without missing a beat, I looked her square in the eye and replied, "Well it wasn't the most fun I've had with my pants down, but it was not too bad!" ☺ She burst out laughing and looked at me and said, "You have the best attitude!" I left them smiling.

This past round of chemo was exceptionally difficult. I ended up admitted to hospital for three days with low electrolytes and heart issues. It's been a teary week. Mentally I am quite drained from the constant pain and stress of it all, but I continue to plow through. People, again I say, make your health and peace of mind your #1 priority so you don't have to go through this beast! Love to you all!

♡☺♡☺♡☺♡☺♡

I had more blood tests two days before chemo Round #4, and miraculously, my potassium and neutrophils and all the other things that had been out of whack managed to revert well enough that we were told we could proceed with the next round. I was filled with dread. I had only been out of the hospital a little over a week, and during that time I was already back in for a chemo consult, tattoos, the CT, information meetings, and had had more blood work as the usual protocol for chemo prep. I didn't know which end was up and was certainly not prepared for more pain and stress with the usual IV challenges and awful physical reactions I continued to have each time.

With one day left before the next chemo, I had to really dig deep to find the strength to go ahead. I set my alarm for another early rise and another long day. Yet again, I had another fitful sleep, anxiously willing my mind to believe that chemo was "good for me" as it killed the cancer cells. Unfortunately, chemo also kills healthy, normal, "fast-growing" cells, hence the hair loss and mouth sores, to name a few reactions—hard evidence that the chemo is indeed in there, working its "magic."

May in Nova Scotia does not always feel like spring, but the morning of chemo Round #4 was indeed spring-like with warm temperatures and birds calling their early greetings to one another. I would've given anything to just curl up on my deck with a big blanket to listen to the beautiful sounds of nature. It was the crack of dawn, and once more, I got wearily into the car. I put my barely packed bag on my lap; the plan was to just sleep the entire day during chemo.

We arrived after an uneventful drive, and this time for some reason I was brought to a different end of the Cancer Centre. We practically had our own room. There was only one other couple in there. Mike was able to get a slightly more comfortable chair. They worked and worked on my arm for several minutes, and finally, after three painful pokes and digs, they got the needle in. I was still worried about another reaction like Round #2 and was also now dealing with PTSD from the potassium horror I had very recently suffered through.

Somehow I got through another long day of chemo infusions, and I stepped out into sparkly daylight, happy that summer was coming soon. Mike and I both really needed warm weather and sunshine, and I was relieved that I was into radiation next and wouldn't have another round of chemo for about eleven weeks.

I never fully grasped the true depth of the term "warrior" when describing a cancer survivor until my own diagnosis and journey. Now, I *completely* understand. A cancer warrior possesses at the very *least*, the following qualities: fierce mental strength to push through some of the darkest hours of their life; mental clarity to keep straight the hundreds of appointments, medical information, tracking, discussions, major decisions and meetings;

courage and tenacity to arrive week after week, round after round, for blood work, CT scans, emergency trips, hospital admissions, IVs, radiation and chemo itself; physical strength to endure, process, and recover from hit after hit after merciless hit with some of the most powerful and toxic of substances entering the human body, and lastly, huge emotional strength not to have a nervous breakdown through it all. I have earned the right to loudly scream, "I am a warrior!" and I am the strongest person I know.

This most honourable designation doesn't come without its disadvantages, though; the aftermath of earning this heavyweight title has left me emotionally destroyed and deeply wounded on all counts.

In the days that followed this last round, I again pushed hard to avoid another hospital admission and worked determinedly to get as much water, supplements, electrolytes, and nourishing food in me as I possibly could while still being completely bedridden, severely in pain, weak, and dizzy upon standing. The cancer battle truly does take many hands to support the journey, and I am forever grateful to all of my family and friends who continually arrived with herbal teas, casseroles, soups, soaps, body creams, and lots of other caring treats as Mike and I continued to unravel. To the world outside of our home, we tried our best to hide the awful devastation we experienced daily, but behind our closed doors, the cancer toll was quite evident to us both as we became more and more worn down. We were now entering the fourth consecutive month of intense pain and overwhelming suffering.

30

GUITAR LADIES AND THE GREATEST GIFT

Planting Day, May 28

When I left my music teaching position in the public school system roughly ten years ago, I decided to open a private studio to teach guitar to adult women. I wanted to be able to teach people in my own home with whom I felt safe and could trust. I began a "word of mouth, recommendations only" music business. What evolved very quickly was a large group of women that I came to love dearly and thoroughly enjoyed. We soon built upon our growing friendships with music recitals, guitar parties, potluck dinners, and trips away. A bond formed that I am most certain will last a lifetime. During my illness, these women rallied together and supported me on a large wave that I rode long and hard. They lifted me up, nurtured me, cared for and loved me at my absolute worst; they checked in with me on a weekly, and for some, daily, basis.

These guitar friends (now a much larger group than when I first began teaching guitar), paired with my besties which I've known and loved for more than twenty-five years, have gifted me the most incredible seed I could grow—my own self-worth. I am eternally grateful for all of these wonderful women, as well as all of my many social media friends. Never before in my life have I felt so cherished and loved by so many. It gave me the strength, joy, and courage needed to continue fighting the fight.

Summer was coming; it would be the first for us in our new home. On a good day if I was out of bed, I was excited to see what flowers would spring up on the property. I knew planting season was approaching, and I wondered if I would have any energy at all to be enjoying the outdoors.

One day my dear friend Marianne asked me how she might be of help. "Do you need anything?" she so sweetly inquired. I chuckled and told her I still had a freezer full of casseroles and a log column in my kitchen with over seventy-five "Get Well" cards attached and overflowing. The cards made me smile, and I felt much encouragement from seeing them. I had so many cards in fact, that I wondered if I needed to start a second column. Marianne replied, "I was reading this article the other day about how to help people going through cancer. It suggested that when people already have plenty of cards, soups, and casseroles, that one should think outside of the obvious. I want to support you, but what can I actually do to help cheer you up?"

What a great question! People really don't ask this question enough of one another. With heartfelt gratitude, I said I would get back to her. I began to think. I had been through so much. *What would make me happy that cannot be acquired or made?* What I truly wanted (and very much needed) was not really tangible; I wanted my hair back, my heartache gone, my worry to diminish, and my pain to dissipate. I wanted peace of mind and promised good health. In short, I wanted my life back.

Was there actually anything that would bring me joy that could be given or purchased? I thought a while longer and then called her back.

"I would like a shrub."

"Hmm," she said. "What kind of shrub?"

"I would like something that I can nurture and grow, something to enjoy for years to come. It doesn't really matter what."

Marianne sounded quite excited and proclaimed, "I'm not going to give you a shrub. I'm going to give you a whole garden! Give me a few days; I'm going to do this for you, Andrea. I will organize something with all of the guitar ladies! I'm so excited! It's going to be great!"

And just like that, she was on it. She sent out many emails and organized the logistics around the whole thing. Between the two of us, we decided I would benefit from what we called "The Healing Garden." I could tend to it each day when I felt better, or I could just go out and sit by it and watch it grow. It would serve as a daily reminder that I was very much loved and supported by a wonderful group of friends. I was grateful for Marianne's kindness and efforts.

Sure enough, several weeks later when it was finally warm enough in our little coastal province to plant delicate, pretty flowers and blooming shrubs, "Planting Day" arrived. This was just five days after chemo Round #4.

It was nine thirty a.m. and Marianne and another dear friend, Karen, arrived with an entire carload full of plants. I couldn't believe my eyes. Karen popped open the hatchback of her Subaru and I saw that it was overflowing with vibrant flowers in pinks, blues, some variegated leaves, numerous plants, and many shrubs. I was in awe.

"These are from your guitar ladies!" Karen announced and Marianne looked at me with a face filled with absolute joy. Marianne had organized the collecting of the plants from all of the women while Karen had gone through her own incredible garden snipping and digging up lots of extra perennials as well. I watched as they unloaded lilac trees, hydrangeas, lilies, hostas, bee balm, echinacea cone flower, daisies, bleeding hearts, pink dianthus, rose peonies, impatiens, Solomon's seal, and much more! They even brought bags of soil and wood chips. All in all, there were fifty-odd plants and shrubs ready for their new home. I was floored. I could not fathom the effort it took to pull this all together. They stood there smiling, Karen in her garden overalls and Marianne with her gloves and trowel.

I was overjoyed to see my dear friends, and I wanted very much to try and watch the progress. I staggered to the outdoor lounge chair, my heart pounding from the effort (even at a snail's pace) and from the strain of just being upright. Obviously I couldn't lift a finger to help them. I felt uncomfortable just sitting and watching them work, but at this point so soon after chemo, I was lucky to be up at all.

They reassured me that this was their gift to me and that I was *supposed* to just sit there, in my teak chaise lounge, letting them do their work. I felt terribly useless and I was humbled by their words of love.

It was an exceptionally hot day, and the two of them worked hard for about six hours, directly in the scorching sun. Up and down on their knees, digging, lugging, shovelling, hosing, and organizing—they didn't stop. Mike dug out an entire garden bed of heavily impacted soil and hoed and cleared another garden bed full of overgrown weeds and stagnant growing bushes. He too was working hard and covered in sweat.

By mid-afternoon, sun still beaming, they announced they were all finished and that it was time for the great reveal. I had been watching them working away all day at two gardens to my left, but I could not see around the corner to the garden bed on the right, which was the truly special one they were proudest of and that had the most colour.

Karen had amazing gardens in her own home in the city and had carefully planned what plants would go where and what was suitable in my coastal environment. It took her several hours to map it all out before planting day came, so I was excited to see what she had come up with in this most special of the garden beds.

"Okay!" they called. "Come see!"

Sweating and weak, wobbly with my walking stick, I came around the corner and was simply awestruck. Pinks, purples, magentas, blues, and whites, all placed so beautifully and carefully together in a bed that measured fifteen feet wide and several feet in depth. It was spectacular.

Tears of gratitude rolled down my face, and my lips started quivering. A huge sob came from me and I started full-out crying. "Oh my gosh!" I whispered. "I love it. It's so beautiful!" They stood there smiling back at me, soil-stained, breathing hard, and covered in sweat. They were both thoroughly exhausted and looked so very satisfied. "I will have this for years to come! And every time I see it I will feel the joy from your love. As I get stronger, I will tend to it and nurture it and watch it grow!" I declared. This, truly, was the greatest gift.

Another dear friend, Sue, who had planned to be a part of the garden crew, had woken up that morning to find she had a flat tire. She was disappointed to have missed the planting and had decided that she would get a sign for the healing garden. Weeks later, when I was sleeping over at her place in the city for an early morning radiation appointment, we sat and looked through various sites to pick out a custom-designed, wrought iron sign. I envisioned "Healing Garden. Est. 2023." She promptly ordered a customized sign, and a month later she showed up at my place with a package. As I opened it, I started crying tears of gratitude and joy all over again. We carefully placed the sign out with the blooming plants. "Look at that! Now it's complete!" What a wonderful, perfect gift. My dearly beloved guitar ladies mean the world to me.

Three days after the healing garden was planted, I decided to give another update to my online family, as I was working away at recovery from chemo round #4.

Social Media Post #12
May 31

Hi peeps!

A little humour today. A friend from away was checking in and asked me how I'm doing. Below was my honest reply:

Hola!! How am I doing? Hmmm . . . . Well, I'm fat, pale, bald, and bedridden! I smell bad, I have diarrhea, and I pee all over myself as the chemo has dried me out soo much even my urine stream is messed up! I have furry teeth from chemo toxins, orange pee, and a chronic heart rate of about 120–150, which makes me faint and gasp for air just going from bed to toilet. I have nightly sweats, insomnia, a dry face, dry peeling feet and no desire to get dressed. I have nausea, headaches from toxins and morphine withdrawal, back pain and sores in my mouth.

Other than that . . . I'm good! ☺

Point being, I'm still smiling, my husband still makes me laugh, I'm still super grateful for my friends and family, and y'all are uplifting me. Life is what it is and I continue to look for the positives. I hope someday I'll have these posts pop up as memories and I'll truly be proud of all that I've overcome. ☺ Radiation starts in a few weeks. 27 sessions. ♡

31

SCAN FOR RAD

I was scheduled to have another CT scan a week before the radiation was to start. This information was to greater assess tissue depth, damage, and any other info inside my pelvis that would help the oncology team prepare for the treatments. I was worried however, as it was only two weeks after my last round of chemo and I was still feeling weak and in pain.

The scan involved an oral contrast medium called Gastrografin that I would need to prepare and drink. Mike came home one evening with the product as well as four typed papers that I was instructed to read. "Gosh," I exclaimed. "This seems a little over the top." There were several pages on when to prepare it, when to drink it, and the potential reactions. Naturally, I felt a little dread at this point, wondering how my body would accept yet another unusual thing thrown at it. I willed myself once again to try to just imagine this liquid as helpful, important, and healing.

Instructions were to drink two teaspoons of the Gastrografin mixed with 300 ml of water. The first dose was any time after eight o'clock the evening before the exam with nothing to eat after midnight. The next dose was two hours before the exam time, and the last dose would be at the hospital, instructed by the nurse.

I mixed up the preparation and chugged it down. It was awful. My nose automatically crinkled and my tongue started to recoil as I swallowed. (It's a lot to chug 300 ml of something one does not like.) "Ugh," I said, breathless and panting as I slammed the glass down on the table. "That was dis-GUSTING!" I could feel my stomach gurgle and swoosh as a slight wave of nausea passed over me. A few minutes later, I felt even worse and decided I should just go to bed.

It was storming and windy that night. I could hear the surf smashing against the shoreline, and it was hard to sleep. I was a little worried about the scan the next morning; yet again, I was expecting and dreading another IV issue with the procedure.

My alarm went off at five thirty. I quickly got out of bed as I was already wide awake. Upon standing I felt even more woozy and nauseated than my usual. I carefully got dressed and fed Duey a very early breakfast as we had to leave at six for a seven o'clock arrival at the hospital.

The drive in was rainy, windy, and again, stressful, as cars zipped and veered around each other in the morning commute. I was still feeling gurgly and nauseated, clutching my next installment of Gastrografin in my mason jar. I was watching the clock and waiting for the exact time to chug-a-lug the next 300 ml. When the dreaded time arrived, Mike pulled over on the highway. I chugged it down. I stopped halfway as my stomach lurched and my mouth became watery. I was breathless as I uttered, "I think I'm going to vomit." Mike looked at me in concern, not just because the thought of me vomiting in the car was unpleasant, but also because we were not sure if vomiting up the important liquid would then muck up the scan.

"Hold it down as best you can," he encouraged, with a nervous smile. With all my might I did my darndest to swallow the rest of it.

"This is not good," I proclaimed. I looked around for a container, anything to use as a barf bag, and realized my only choice would be back in the mason jar. *Good lord, that would be a challenge. The diameter is a lot tinier than a toilet bowl.* Somehow, miraculously, I held on and we managed a vomit-free car ride.

"Good morning, Andrea!" A young nurse smiled as she greeted me in the waiting room.

"Hi there," I replied. I smiled as brightly as I could as another wave of nausea suddenly washed over me.

"You drank the preparation last night and again this morning?" she asked.

"I did, yes, but I am really, *really* queasy. I can't drink the last of it. I'm honestly just trying my hardest to keep down what I already drank. I'm sorry."

"Oh gosh, don't worry," she reassured me. "I'll speak with radiology and see if we can skip the last dose."

Instantly my body relaxed. I was so very happy to learn that this was even an option.

I waited with Mike in the waiting room. There was a family sitting across from us; we were practically touching knees we were crammed in so closely. I was wishing I had brought my wig or at least my hat, as I now felt quite exposed, awkward, and embarrassed for Mike. I knew people would look at him with pity. *Aw, poor man with the sick, bald wife. What a shame.* (I had seen the looks before and knew them well.) I had felt too sick in the dark, wee hours of the morning to put on my wig or to even remember a hat; I was just trying to get out of the house on time.

"Good news!"

I turned and saw the nurse coming back toward me.

"You don't have to drink the last bit. We will try to get the info we need without it."

"Okay, great," I said. "Also, you need to know that my veins are extremely small and people have a hard time getting the needles in for IVs and blood work." I smiled at her, feebly. "I would love to have your best 'needler.'"

"No problem! We are all good here, don't you worry," Nurse Cheery replied.

I sat back down and did my best not to projectile-vomit all over the family still sitting across from us. I started sweating as the nausea took over. I looked at Mike. *He must see me as just so pathetic.* I was quite the sight—pale, sweating, feeling horrid, bald as an egg, and rocking back and forth, trying my hardest to keep myself together, but yet again, crying quietly.

"Okay, my dear, we are all set." A nurse came and took my arm and guided me to the next area to get the IV prepped.

It was a small room with a big La-Z-Boy. I was familiar with it, as it was the same kind of chair in the chemo centre. "Okay, just sit back and try to relax." She sat down on the stool and looked at my arms. "Hmm." She sighed. "Hmm." She sighed again. She then carried her stool to my other side and started looking again. "Hmm. Hmm. Hmm." She got up with her stool once more and went back to my left arm. "I'll be right back. I'm going to get my vein finder."

She returned after a few minutes with a little laser-type machine that shows all of the veins in the arms, not unlike Mike's laser stud-finder we use on the walls at home. She held the vein finder over my arms. It would have been quite fascinating for me to see had I not been scared and still trying hard not to vomit.

"Oh wow. You really *don't* have much to work with, do you. These veins are tiny!" She seemed surprised, even with my warnings only moments earlier.

"Yup," *deep breath*, "just what I was telling you." I quietly mumbled.

"Okay. Well. I think I got one." She began the procedure of tourniquet, slapping my arm, applying rubbing alcohol, and then a poke.

A sharp pain. "Ouch!" I yelled, surprising both of us.

"Oh my gosh, I am so sorry!"

She had blown through my vein. She looked so surprised. I just looked straight ahead, clenching my teeth and trying to breathe deeply. "Are you okay? I was sure that was a good one." She looked genuinely startled.

"I'm okay," I replied, holding back tears. "It's not your fault."

"Yes, but I really don't like hurting you." Her empathy made it even harder to maintain my brave facade. "I'm going to try again, and then if I can't get it I will get my supervisor, okay?"

"Okay."

She tried again.

"Ow!" I jumped. She jumped. I think I was about to give her an anxiety attack.

"I'll be right back. My supervisor is really, really good at this, and she will get it in no problem. Are you okay if I leave you for a minute?"

I lied and said yes. I was actually just seconds away from power puking; fully locked and very much loaded.

She left and I immediately had a horrible wave of nausea pass over me with such ferocity I knew it could not be held in check. I started seeing black tunnels. I was now completely covered in sweat from bald head to slippered toe. There was no garbage can that I could readily see. I tried to gain control, but my body powerfully launched itself into full evacuation mode and I violently threw up. Piles and piles of liquid expelled all over the floor, the chair, and on me as my body repeatedly convulsed. I started to faint. I was still upright in the chair and was concerned I would fall forward and break my nose. I called loudly for help. I was still seeing black tunnels and panting when after what seemed like forever, the supervisor walked in.

"Oh my heavens!" she exclaimed. Hurriedly, she stepped in the vomit puddles and squeezed between the wall and the La-Z-Boy to get behind me to tilt the chair back, raising my feet. She ran out and ran back with cold cloths, placing them on my forehead, my neck, and my wrists. *These people really are not paid enough.*

"Are you doing okay?" she asked.

I had a horrible taste in my mouth and was seeing stars, but at least my tummy felt better. I looked up at her, eyes still watering. "Yes, I'm okay."

She smiled. "Oh, you poor thing."

She found another nurse and they cleaned up the mess, gave me fresh robes and gave me several more minutes to calm down. I was secretly wishing at this point they would just send me home.

"Okay, I'm going to get this needle in so we can get this done and get you outta here." She patted my arm and smiled at me. I was too exhausted to react and so I just laid there, drool coming from my mouth, staring off into space.

She looked at my arms, without the vein finder, and to my astonishment, got the needle in on the first try and I barely felt it. "Ta da!" she sang out. I looked down and there it was, the needle in all its glory, in my arm and ready to go.

"You are amazing!" I cried. "I'm so grateful for you!" I was astounded. When you least expect it, sometimes things actually go well.

"Okay, when you're ready, we will go get this done." She stood there, looking down at me in my weak, miserable mess.

I took a big breath. "Okay," I mumbled, "let's do this."

She helped me up and I walked down the hall, shaking, sweating, and trying to regain my composure. I walked right past Mike. He didn't see me and I realized he was likely oblivious to my whole ordeal, absorbed in his own work on his computer and most likely multi-tasking.

In the scan room, I was greeted by three very kind female technicians. They helped me onto the scan table and explained the procedure, to which I politely told them this was about my sixth time and I was prepared for them to start. The dye was injected, I did my thing, and was finished in a matter of minutes.

"Okay, great job. You just take your time getting up and we will walk you out."

To my surprise, I started crying again. "I'm really sorry. It's been a rough couple of months and I just need a minute."

Their faces showed much empathy and they looked like they wanted to hug me.

After a few minutes, I pulled it together, got up, and walked back to get my clothes bag next to Mike. I stooped low to collect the handles on the bag and sniffed loudly as my nose was still running and I was still crying. Mike looked up at me and was a little taken aback at how rough I looked.

"Is everything okay?" he asked.

"Yes," I replied, trying my best again not to have a complete meltdown right there. Hands shaking, I grabbed my clothes and hobbled off to the change room. The nurse removed my IV and I changed quickly into my still damp vomit clothes. I came out, found Mike, and through gritted teeth said, "We need to go, fast. I am *this* close to having a nervous breakdown." I pinched my thumb and index finger together and you couldn't even see a space. "Just please get me in the car."

Without a word, Mike packed up his stuff and we walked as swiftly as I was capable down the long hallway. To our surprise we heard familiar voices say, "Hey you guys!" and I looked up and saw Jo and Hans, Mike's aunt and her husband, all smiles. They jumped up and moved toward us; they were surprised and so glad to see us. Jo was there for a casting and assessment for an injured wrist. I kept walking and hung on to Mike's arm. They saw my face, the tears, the defeat, and of course, my very bald egg head.

I retreated behind Mike, still shaking and crying, and mumbled, "I really can't talk right now; we need to go."

I'm certain they were quite unnerved by my feeble, emotional appearance and perhaps worried that I'd just received deadly news or something. I heard Mike say, "I'll call you later and explain," and we quickly left.

All self-control gone, I got into the car and let loose another long, horrible, moaning cry. Tears of frustration and exhaustion rolled down my face, like a river had broken through a dam. Another seemingly run-of-the-mill procedure gone horribly wrong. My spirit was *completely* crushed.

32

THE BIG, BAD VAGINAL DILATOR

Lara has a house here in Nova Scotia, and annually she and her husband, their two daughters, and their two dogs make the long trek home from California to spend quality time with friends and family. I wasn't sure if she was coming back again after having just travelled all this way and back only a month earlier on her solo visit. To my complete joy she arrived home again in June, family and dogs in tow, and even though she was busy with her own family this time, she continued her visits and care.

One day when she was visiting, I got an odd phone call. I didn't recognize the number. "Hello?" I answered, feeling tired of always getting calls and information at this point.

"Andrea?" A male voice, with a heavy accent. "This is radiation department calling. I am Dr. So-and-So."

I sat right up, listening carefully now, as I had been waiting for this call. I was expecting to receive the dates and information needed to start radiation. My heart pounded; I was so very worried about this aspect of the treatments.

"Do you have pen and paper to write things down? Very, very important."

"Yes. I am ready, go ahead."

"Do you have sexual partner?"

"Pardon?"

"Do you have sexual partner to keep the vagina working?"

Oh my God. "Uh, I have a husband, if that's what you're asking?"

"Are you having the regular intercourse with husband?"

"Uh, not at the moment, no. I just had a hysterectomy not too long ago, and I'm going through chemo." *Awkward…*

"Okay. You need to have the sexual intercourse three times a week with the partner, or you can buy vaginal dilator."

"Uh, okay…. What is that? And…why?"

"It is extremely, extremely important to have sexual relations with your husband or a dilator after the radiation ceases. You need to read about vaginal stenosis."

"Uh, vaginal what?"

"Stenosis. Stenosis of the vagina."

"…Okay…"

"You must begin the sexual intercourse two weeks after radiation, or vagina will shrink."

Good Lord! What? "Um, alright…?"

"So, will you be getting the dilator or using the husband for the vagina?"

"Uh, the hus—…m-my husband for th— m-my vagina."

"Okay, Andrea, that is very, very good. You can start the sexual intercourse after the radiation. Okay? Questions?"

I was completely blank on that front. "Uh, no. No, I understand."

"Okay. Very Good. We'll speak again in a few weeks about radiation, okay?"

"Okay, yup, yes. Yes. Okay. I mean…yes, sounds good. Thank you!"

I hung up. Lara and Mike were waiting in the other room. "What was *that* all about?" Lara asked, looking entertained and curious.

"Uh…my vagina?" I answered. I had heard the word over the phone more in those five minutes than I had heard in my entire life.

She burst out laughing. "What do you mean?" she asked, sitting right up, ready to try and understand this crazy conversation.

And so it went. I explained the conversation in between hysterical fits of giggles.

We looked up vaginal stenosis and were astounded to learn that the vagina can and does shrink.

"What?' Lara said, shocked. "It can really shrink?" We were both amazed. In some cases, it is irreversible. Future relations with a partner and any medical procedures with a speculum can become extremely painful. It can destroy a person's self-esteem.

"Boy," Lara said, still half chuckling, "it's good to know that Nova Scotia Health really cares about women's vaginas!"

And so, after much thought, I diligently went to the hospital drugstore, had a very awkward conversation with a young pharmacist, purchased a five-piece, hot-pink dilator kit, and made a mental note to make sure I used it.

33
RADIATION AND MARINA

Not long after the dilator purchase I looked at my calendar and saw that June 13th was quickly approaching. In bright red marker I'd written "Rad Day" in my day-planner and I'd circled it three times. *Ha.* I sighed. *Like there was any chance I'd miss that . . .* it was the only thing on my mind and the glaring sight of the red ink against the stark white paper made me *beyond* anxious.

In the days leading up to these next treatments I realized I still didn't know what to expect. I felt quite scared at the thought of being "microwaved" every day for almost twenty minutes. The appointment a few weeks back to discuss radiation in detail was only a very brief meeting with a nurse who emphatically reviewed the importance of the dilator to commence two weeks after the last day of treatment. I was not yet fully aware at that point that the effects of radiation would be long-lasting, far-reaching, and entirely worrisome.

Soon enough, the dreaded radiation day arrived. I was still recovering from the last round of chemo twenty days prior and the more recent, nasty experience with the Gastrografin. I felt incredibly feeble. I was paler than pale (even for a redhead), and I walked hunched over like an ailing, arthritic ninety-year-old. To say I was struggling was an understatement. Feeling beyond worn out, I continued to fight, but now, only on autopilot.

We arrived at the Cancer Centre and checked in. The radiation unit was located just around the corner from the usual oncology checkup location. The lady at the reception desk was unpleasant and made very little eye contact; cancer patients deserve better! I wanted and desperately needed a cheery face, as this was all so new to me and I was full of fear.

I registered and was handed a piece of paper with the appointment times for the rest of the week. I asked if these were set times and the same for the next five weeks and was told that they vary from week to week and that sometimes an appointment can be changed, even within twenty-four hours. This made it really tricky for Mike to schedule driving and sitting with me as he was still handling work meetings, IT support, conference calls, and on-call requests from his team.

After the paperwork was complete, I was instructed to go around the corner to change into a johnnie shirt and robe. I did so and noticed that my arms were so weak, even carrying out my bag of clothes was difficult. After five long months in bed, I had developed severe muscle atrophy and could not carry anything heavier than a small purse or my phone. Only a year before, I had the strength to hold our two-hundred-pound dog back in his moments of lunging and rearing. I took a deep breath and walked into the waiting room, my eyes searching for Mike. From our many months in the chemo waiting room, this new place seemed somewhat familiar—a bunch of ill-looking people, some bald like me, and most with a partner or a friend accompanying them. I sat down, heart pounding, and waited fretfully.

I took in my surroundings, trying to acclimatize to my new routine for the next five weeks. There were several different hallways that led to the main reception area, and I kept hearing laughter all around me from various staff members and patients alike. Laughter is such a wonderful thing. It always perks a creature up to hear a joyful, spirited person, and I wondered if this laughter belonged to a staff member in the radiation department. One particular laugh seemed consistent with each of the groups I saw. My eyes looked for the face that belonged to the joyfulness I could hear.

"Andrea?" A smiling, young tech in matching green pants and shirt stood with her hands in her pockets, looking at me.

"Yes?" My voice sounded scared.

"Hi there, I'm Marina. How are you doing?"

God love her, she asked me how I'm doing! I was feeling quite nervous and I told her that.

"Aw, I understand. We are going to take good care of you, I promise. And I'll accompany you to the radiation room and back. Are you okay to walk with me?"

I couldn't believe how kind she was. "I think so. I have tachycardia when I stand up, so I just need a minute." I was wary of hospitals and all of the various personalities I had encountered at this point, yet Marina seemed sincere and caring, and I desperately needed a comforting, patient person. Her smile was so reassuring; I couldn't help but feel safe.

She waited while I carefully stood up, finding my balance. My heart began to race and I instantly had pressure and ringing in my ears with some light dizziness. I grabbed the nearby rail and needed another minute. I hated making her wait, but I didn't have a choice. After a bit, things settled down.

"Okay. I'm ready." I looked at Mike. He gave me an "off you go" sort of look. Marina reached out to support me and kept her arm firmly linked through mine the entire walk down yet another long hallway. "I'm sorry, I get really dizzy these days. I really appreciate your help."

She patted my hand as we walked. "Oh, that's okay. That's what we're here for. We want to keep you super safe as you come and go down our hall-ways." She spoke joyfully and I knew that indicated she loved people and enjoyed her job.

I said something funny then and she laughed loudly. *It was her! The beautiful laughing human. She* was responsible for the happiness and laughter all around us. My heart filled with joy and I felt truly grateful to meet her and make this connection. She didn't seem much older than my daughters, but I was amazed at how mature she was, working in this very important job. She kept up a friendly conversation as we walked down the hallway, and I instantly felt like we were old friends just catching up and chatting away.

We arrived at the radiation room. It was dimly lit and two other rad techs were there. "Are you Andrea?" one asked.

"That's me." I now felt a teeny bit happier and maybe a smidgeon more brave. They introduced themselves and asked details like when my birthday was, etc.

"Okay. You need to take off your robe and get up on the table. Once you're up, you need to lower your underwear down a bit and we will get you into position using your rad tattoos. The whole procedure will only take about twenty minutes or so, okay?"

"Okay," I replied.

I got up on the table, they wriggled and adjusted me, and then in I went, arms overhead and music playing. I was still mostly terrified, but at least I felt like I could trust them and that they would be good to me. My heart pounded as the large machines slowly rotated around my torso. Green laser lines bounced on the ceiling. I had been so traumatized by constant, unexpected pain over the last several months that I assumed this would really hurt. I held my breath over and over as the machines turned and moved all around me. I felt thoroughly vulnerable. It was a long twenty minutes as my adrenalin pumped and my muscles clenched. I repeatedly tried to relax as I listened to the music quietly playing. Subsequently the techs came back in, pulled the bed out of the machine, and announced the session was all finished. I let out a huge sigh. I was very relieved that I didn't experience intense pain on that first day.

By day three I'd figured out that my radiation sessions were roughly the length of four or five songs, and I mentally kept track and counted each song as it played. I knew I would be done soon and found the music very helpful. The machines all sounded alike and moved in similar fashion each time, so I came to quickly anticipate when they would be finished. Each time I was done, the upbeat techs would come in and say, "Great job, Andrea, you're all done for today."

"Yay!" I'd say, or, "Whoo hoo!"

You may be wondering if there is any preparation needed prior to each radiation treatment. There is, and it's pretty straightforward. With pelvic radiation you need to have the exact same bladder size each and every time. If it's too empty, the radiation can damage the internal organs. If it's too full, it's not accurately reaching where it needs to go to keep the continuity.

I was instructed to empty my bladder forty-five minutes before the radiation time and then to immediately drink 500 ml of water. The chugging of water was the easy part, I simply set my alarm and drank from my measured water bottle when the alarm went off. The emptying of the bladder part was not so easy. We lived forty-five minutes away. With parking being difficult and occasional work on the highways or car accidents jamming the route, we knew we had to consistently leave *more* than fifty minutes before my appointment, which meant I couldn't pee at home. It meant I had to plan my route to the minute of locating and using an available bathroom, and it quickly became a logistical nightmare. We stopped at various gas stations, coffee shops, McDonalds, Canadian Tire, a fabric store, and even at more obscure places on occasion.

One day, because we'd left in a bit of a hurry, I hadn't bothered to wear my hat, although I was now rarely seen without one. My wig was just too hot to wear now that it was late June and my big, boofy beach hat hid my baldness quite well. We left the house and bombed along in our little sports car. My pee alarm went off as we cruised down the highway and I knew we needed to pull in to the nearest gas station. I looked around for something to put on my head; I'd forgotten I would need to stop in public. With no options, I sighed heavily. I was going to have to brave going in to the public gas station with my big ole, shiny bald head. I was *really* bald at this point, not even a spriglet on top—bald like a freshly birthed chicken egg!

I got out of the car and faked confidence as I walked in wearing my giant Elton John sunglasses, a bright blue sundress, my jean jacket, and wedge sandals. It was obvious I was a female, but with my bald head, people were staring, trying to figure out what my deal was. Embarrassed and flustered, my brain mixed up the bathroom signs.

Hurriedly I yanked open the bathroom door to what I thought was the women's. Rushing now, as I was about to burst, I quickly locked the door behind me, turned, and then took in the very dirty bathroom. There was urine on the floor, toilet paper strewn about, a wall urinal, and a toilet with the seat up. Brown streakers lined the bowl. "Oh dear lord, Andrea, you IDIOT!" I said out loud. I was dancing the squirmy pee dance at this point and had no choice but to swiftly sit on the dirty toilet. Instant relief. I finished, washed up and then quickly walked out of the disgusting bathroom.

As I neared the cash, I saw the same three men in line who'd just watched me race past only moments earlier. The cashier was staring at me again. Given the fact that all four of them had stared at me from the moment I walked in and had watched as I bee-lined it to the back, I was pretty sure they'd all seen me go in to the men's washroom. Well. I marched on past them like I *owned* the place. I could see them whispering and then the cashier threw her hands in the air. I heard her say, "I'm not even gonna ask." Clearly the question was, "Was that a man or a woman?"

Another day, Mike and I set out to get to the radiation appointment, and about a minute after we left our driveway we came to a complete stop. Highway workers were repairing the road from local flooding. The wait was long and I anxiously looked at the clock. "I'm not going to get to the gas station on time!"

Mike looked in the rear-view mirror and quickly solved the problem. "We're going to have to take the other way around," he announced. He did a U-turn, adeptly swinging the car around, and we raced against the clock to get to another gas station. As we flew down the road, my alarm went off. I yelled to him over the music that it was time. "Right now?" he yelled back. "Yes. Right NOW!" He quickly pulled over on the side of the road.

Cars zoomed by us and our little vehicle shook as they passed a little too closely. I ever so carefully stepped out only to discover that the shoulder of the road was eroding. I had no place to even squat. I opened the back door as a visual shield from the other cars and promptly hiked up my dress and emptied my bladder right there in front of my poor husband. (There really is no dignity with this horrible disease.) He searched for some leftover fast food napkins in the console for me to use as toilet paper. It must've been quite a sight for him; me grinning away, my big bald head gleaming in the sun, big black sunglasses on, dress hiked well up to the tops of my thighs, and teetering on the brink of an embankment in high-heeled sandals, almost peeing on my own two feet.

He couldn't help but laugh with me. Cars honked loudly as they drove by, and I held on to the car door handles to keep from falling down the embankment. Hurriedly I wiggled and shook myself and threw the soiled napkins in the ditch. I felt badly for littering but I didn't have any other place to put them. "Thank you, Tim Hortons!" I called into the air as we drove away—they always gave lots of napkins in the drive-thru.

Miraculously, we made it to my appointment with one minute to spare. We were again working hard with each other to make the very best of a difficult situation. Peeing on the side of the road and nearly falling into the ditch with such weakness and ill health really was a preposterous situation. We laughed, seeing the humour of it; a true testament to our friendship and love.

The timing and location for the pre-radiation pee became the main topic of conversation almost the entire summer as I cycled through chugging plenty of water and emptying out the other end. Monday to Friday, Monday to Friday, five long weeks in a row. Sue helped out considerably during this time. She lived near the hospital, and several times each week she would either drive me over, pick me up, sit with me, or host me to spend the night at her house. She cooked lunches and dinners for me. She was a true star, giving me all of her available time. It really made a difference, as driving in and out every day, ninety minutes round trip, five days a week, for five weeks in a row took a lot of time, a lot of energy, and a *lot* of gas.

As the days passed, Marina continued to make sure I got back safely each and every time she was scheduled with me. I was grateful to have her there, and I marvelled at her consistent, upbeat personality. Her light shone brightly, helping every single patient she was with. When I waited in the main area, I always heard her laughter and upbeat attitude before I even saw her. (People who are going through such awful cancer treatments and appointments suffer terribly and desperately need this positivity.) She brought out everyone's best.

One day as I greeted the techs and climbed up on the table, I fondly spoke about my daughters for the umpteenth time. I told them how well the girls were handling everything and how much I loved them. Marina asked how old they were.

"Twenty-four and twenty-two."

"Oh! I am the same age as your older daughter!"

I asked when her birthday was. Lo and behold, it was coming up the very next week. Curiosity took over and I asked what her plans were. She explained that she loved lemon-banana cake and that she and her friends were getting together to make one for her birthday. I had never heard of this combination of cake before; it sounded sort of odd to me but she happily explained it and we had a good laugh as I tried to wrap my head around it. I decided then and there that I would make her a homemade birthday card, and while I was getting my radiation that day I envisioned a colourful card with a yellow border, bright, big bananas and lots of lemons all connected with scrolly black ink.

I started the card as soon as I got home. It took a bit of effort as my hands were stiff and painful, and I got tired of colouring halfway through. I was excited to give her the little card and handwritten message inside about how wonderful she was; she reminded me a lot of my own girls, so truly kind-hearted. I wanted her to feel the same joy that she gave me.

Early on the morning of Marina's birthday I received a call that one of the machines wasn't working and they had to bump me. I was happy that I got an unexpected day off from the microwave but sad that I couldn't bring her card in to her, on her special day. The weekend was coming, which meant it would be Monday before she would receive it. That just *wouldn't* do! I asked Mike to drive her card in anyway and leave it for her as a surprise.

On Monday I was back to radiation, but Marina was not scheduled with me for a few days. Finally, I saw her in the hallway. When she saw me her face lit up with a giant grin. "Thank you for the card! That was so sweet of you." She gave me a huge hug and seemed sincerely touched by my efforts. As much as I wanted radiation to be over, I really enjoyed Marina and I was going to miss her when I was done. I tried to be as kind and as complimentary as I could to her, showing my gratitude for her efforts every day, and I was glad that I could bring a little bit of sunshine to her as well; she worked so hard for everyone else to make their day brighter, I wanted her to know she was invaluable.

With the sessions accumulating, I managed fairly well at first. I was relieved that everyone was as positive as they were; however, even still, I always felt "off" after I finished a treatment. Although the machines were lasers and non-invasive, the radiation itself still made me feel vulnerable and battered, like my sensitive body was in an internal, worked-up electrical state. I frequently cried in the changing room after I was done the session, shaking and holding my head in my hands. I tried my hardest to be quiet, as people all around me were dealing with the same stuff and I didn't want them to feel more discouraged. Sometimes, I would hug myself as I looked in the long mirror. I would talk to myself and say, "Andrea, you're doing great, you really are." But I would cry all over again as a pale, tired, completely bald and broken person looked back at me in the mirror. I didn't recognize this person, and I cried for the girl I no longer saw. I missed her greatly.

To not recognize my own smiling face, day in and day out, a face that had looked back at me for fifty-two years, was another loss and a cause of grief. Daily anxiety paired with sheer exhaustion and the effort it took to be upbeat and positive also led to pent-up emotion in those changing rooms. I was truly broken-hearted, longing for the life I once had and loved so very much. The past several months seemed like an endless, drawn-out nightmare, and I longed to wake up.

After two weeks, the treatments became more physically challenging. The accumulation of the powerful laser treatment on my abdomen was becoming painful, with deep internal aching. My hot, blistering, itchy skin made even simple things like wearing a seatbelt and putting on underwear simply awful. The staff thoughtfully asked me what creams I was using and gave me some helpful tips. When they tucked in the sheets at the lower part of my legs, Marina would pat my limbs, empathizing with my situation and tenderly giving me reassurance that I would be okay.

Because I mostly saw the same staff members each session, I became familiar with all of them. I shared little bits about my life, such as the fact that I was a music teacher, a wife, a mother, and that I have Duey. The staff was so involved with us, a day or two would pass and then I would have the same staff member again and they would ask, "Did Duey enjoy the beach? How is his paw healing? Did your daughter enjoy her visit with you?" Genuine questions engaging me in a way that showed they listened and really cared. I truly felt those staff members in radiation were second to none.

Now, you may already imagine that pelvic radiation is nasty stuff, but it's more than that—it's a complete nightmare. I spent the majority of July and August with severe incontinence and spent most nights hopping up from the dinner table and racing to the bathroom with virtually no warning. Because radiation shrank and inflamed my bladder, my urethral area became very tiny and painful, and I developed acute cystitis. Each and every time I used the toilet, I was in toe-clenching pain. I dreaded having to go to the bathroom and felt stressed and afraid. At one point, the pain was so bad, I requested a urinalysis; for months I was convinced I had an infection. Sadly, no; this was just my new way of life and, quite miserably, remains so.

On the backside, many a dinner was interrupted with my bowels raging. Each and every thing I ate went *right* through me. "Oh for heaven's sake, this is SO ANNOYING!" I'd yell, as, with no warning, I'd hop up and race as quickly as I could to the bathroom, completely embarrassed and frustrated. "There she goes!" Mike would call lovingly from the table. (I had a few occasions in those months where I considered wearing an adult diaper as I was so afraid of having accidents when travelling to my appointments.)

It was suggested by a family member that radiation was a little reprieve from chemo and "not so bad." Naively, I had envisioned feeling strong and gaining in health, yet evolving complications—severe and inconsistent pelvic floor dysfunctions which emerged quickly and were unexpected at the best of times, and the embarrassing incontinence—forced me to continue to spend the next two months holed up in my home. The radiation appointments themselves were all I basically risked stepping out for.

Shockingly, the radiation also shrank my "private exterior bits" down to more than *half* their size. Imagine that for a moment. Radiation shrinks *everything*. It was nerve wracking each time I had a bath and discovered parts were still shrinking and well beyond my control. My quality of life in all pelvic departments has been horribly affected. I attend pelvic physio every week, trying desperately to recover. In addition, I have constant discomfort in my hips from bone-density loss.

After the fourteenth round of external pelvic radiation, the day came for the dreaded brachytherapy; a session of internal, vaginal radiation. Out of all my treatments, I feared this the most. It would be an extremely awkward procedure, and I was very nervous thinking about it. Even though this was five months' post-hysterectomy, I was still having a great deal of tenderness and pain inside and did not want any more additional discomfort. I was also still plagued by nasty, angry, external hemorrhoids from the seven-pound clay baby from hell that nearly destroyed me. Feeling stressed out and afraid for this next treatment, my cortisol levels went up exponentially as the date neared. I tried to be calm but to no avail.

The day finally came for the brachytherapy appointment, and I met with another group of rad techs as we reviewed the entire process. The radiation "wand" was prepared with a computer system to accommodate each patient personally. Imagine! A "custom-made" dildo. I had to lie as still as possible as they slowly inserted it, and I felt pain and discomfort right away. My knees shook and my back ached as I tried my hardest to stay in the correct position. Having this object inside, attached to a machine, was nerve-wracking in and of itself, and *hugely* emotional.

It brought painful memories from my invasive, raw biopsy, the fear, pain and complications from the hysterectomy, the years of suffering from endometriosis and severe bleeding, and many more emotional experiences that my body had held onto. Laying there, exhausted and sore, I felt beyond vulnerable and became extremely upset. I ended up quietly sobbing. It was a long thirteen minutes on the table, alone in the room, with no music playing this time to help me count it down. I tried to run through four songs in my head, as a way of figuring out when I would be done. Finally finished, the techs came in and removed the wand. I was quite shaken and still very emotional. Silent tears continued to stream down my face; tears of pain, fear, relief, anxiety, fatigue, and long-held suffering. The nurses and techs were very good with me as I tried to explain my emotions. They gently shared that my reaction was common and that women hold much trauma in this delicate area of their bodies.

I cleaned myself up and ambled out. Mike met me in the hallway, and, no longer able to hold back, I audibly sobbed and shook in his arms. It was comforting to know he understood and that I didn't need to say anything more.

We made yet another long drive home to our place of solitude and I realized (as life sped by with the endless treatments) that I hadn't updated my friends in a while. I wrote the following:

Social Media Post #13
July 14

Hey peeps!! I'm here!!! ♡ Still alive. ☺ (Many of you have asked me that lately.) I've been sort of checked out as my cancer journey continues and I'm just soo drained. I've been doing the pelvic radiation lately. Oh boy, what a treat. I've gone in to the Cancer Centre at the Victoria General Hospital five days a week for the past month. I've had 22 sessions so far. Each day I climb onto a table and get zapped for about 20 or so minutes per session. It has left me extremely tired and quite sore (with the yucky complications of my remaining pelvic organs, you'll likely understand why I've been a little AWOL lately). This has dragged on for far too long. But! In the words of Bon Jovi, WHOOOOOOOA . . . I'm half-way there (well, 2/3rds really) Whoooooa!! Living on a prayer!!!! ☺

One silly moment I will share: one day when I was finished the radiation session, I twisted off the table and felt something weird clinging to my underwear. Distractedly, I smiled at the radiation tech, put on my robe and ambled out. I walked down the long hallway, perturbed, as now I had this strange item rubbing on my ankles but when I looked down, I couldn't see anything. Staff in hallways stopped talking as I walked by. When I got to my change room, I burst out laughing as I realized I was dragging an *elephant-sized*, blue pee pad (basically the size of a baby blanket) all the way down the hallway, attached to my underwear!!!!! I bet the techs in the rad room were thinking . . . Now where did that pee pad get to? It was right here a minute ago!! (And I thought toilet paper on my shoe was bad . . . . ☺)

Anyway. I'll be finished all treatments by September. It's been almost 3/4 of a year with pain and stress, but I'm thankful that I can continue to fight this fight and I am blessed with family and friends.

Happy summer y'all!

Love ya ♡

Brachytherapy #1 was followed by seven more sessions of the usual pelvic radiation. I continued with more and more accumulated pain and was barely sleeping at all. Again, like during the post-hysterectomy, I could no longer sleep comfortably on my stomach, and I continued to suffer from deep exhaustion. Thank goodness it was the summer; I ultimately decided to skip the underwear and lived in big billowy dresses so that my skin was less irritated across my abdomen by any sort of waistband.

I pushed through those last few treatments and slowly could see the light at the end the tunnel, counting down the final days to the end of all radiation. I was getting through it, showing up daily, looking forward to being finished with the endless drives, the bathroom stops on the way, and all the water I had to chug.

Of course, looking back, those five weeks seem like a blur. As I think back on my radiation days, my mind replays all of the mishaps during the daily outings—the elephant-sized pee pad stuck to my underwear; the embarrassing moment at the gas station; nearly toppling down the embankment while peeing on the side of the highway; and then, nearing the end of rad treatments, yet another incident.

I needed to get more blood work done, as I needed to prepare for the upcoming chemo round. It was an easy drive as the clinic was just at the end of our highway, so I made the decision to give Mike a break. I hadn't driven in over six months and wanted to feel independent and normal for a brief outing. Even though I was extremely weak, I knew sitting in the car and stepping on the gas pedal was manageable. I had the top down on the sports car, and the music was blasting. At the intersection, a truck pulled up beside me with a pretty girl in the passenger seat. She was checking out the car and then me. I think she must have thought I was a bald, rich, old man. I had a big black sweater on and looked sort of masculine, but then I pulled out my lip gloss and put it on in the rear-view mirror. She got a funny look on her face and they promptly sped off.

As I was driving for another brief outing on another day, a man pulled up beside me. I was wearing my big, boofy hat but then took it off as the wind was picking up and I didn't want it to blow off my head in the convertible. He glanced over and I smiled at him. He saw dress, boobs, jewellery, and my shiny bald head. Same reaction as the girl, days earlier—awkwardness, confusion, disgust. (I'd like to think I made real progress for the trans community in this small little village, looking like a man in women's clothing.) I must say, there were far too many moments that summer where I felt humiliated and sad, and I adjusted and pivoted again and again, trying hard to accept my "new normal."

Finally, the day came when all the external radiation was complete and I had only one last internal session to go. I really dreaded the brachytherapy but at least knew now what to expect. I again found it to be incredibly awkward and painful. With the wand inserted during the treatment, I couldn't fully extend my legs the way I needed to get into the correct position. The techs seemed a little surprised. Brachytherapy was the most damaging to my insides, and in hindsight, the discomfort and pain I experienced during it was likely indicative of the beginning of vaginal stenosis. Now, many months later, I am still dealing with bleeding, pain, badly shrunken parts, and I suffer regularly. I worry and wonder if I will ever fully recover.

Upon completion of the second brachytherapy, radiation was officially over. I was done! Another big box checked off a very lengthy list. I was so grateful for how amazing the rad staff were that I wrote thank-you cards for each of them and shared how much I appreciated all of their efforts. As I handed out the cards, I tearfully said goodbye to Marina and shared again with her that she was exceptional.

As I turned the corner one last time leaving the radiation area, it really sank in that I was *finished*. More happy tears streamed down my face. I wanted to skip down the long hallway, partly because I was overjoyed and partly because they were late starting and I had almost peed everywhere as I handed out the thank-you cards. What I ended up doing was an awkward, half-skip, knees-locked-together, feet-moving-rapidly, squirmy dance all the way down the long hallway, but with minimal fervour as I was still feeling quite weak.

Mike was again waiting for me and this time I fell into his arms with much excitement as we had completed the biggest block of treatments. I wore a grin wider than the Cheshire cat in Alice in Wonderland. "I am so happy to be finished radiation!" I practically yelled this in the changing area. "When we get through the hospital doors will you take my picture outside?" Mike smiled down at me, his relief equaling my joy.

Now I just had two more chemotherapy sessions left (I recalled Dr. Scott describing "the chemo sandwich"—four chemos, twenty-seven radiations, and two more chemos) and then *all* treatments would be over. I was going to crank the bell with much vigour.

Social Media Post #14
July 21

The universe keeps me balanced. Today I cried hard-core-ugly tears of joy as I finished my last radiation session. Then I quickly shimmied down the hallway so I wouldn't pee my pants (ironically they were 30 minutes late getting me started today, of all days). I just made it to the bathroom in time, grateful for no accidents. In my joy and haste to get quickly changed and out of there, I clumsily stabbed myself in the eyeball with my sunglasses while pulling my johnnie shirt over my head.

All this to say that if my life was a movie, Melissa McCarthy would be me, completely bald, grinning from ear to ear in a mint-green hospital gown shuffling as fast as possible down the hallway, knees locked together, trying not to pee, and then playing the clumsy idiot in the changing room. ☺

34

CHEMO ROUND #5

Two weeks to the day after I finished the radiation, I started chemo round #5. They don't mess around with the timelines—no vacation days in this protocol. Turns out, this round was my worst one yet.

I had high hopes that I would be okay in this round, as it had been eleven weeks since my last chemo back in May. I figured this one might go a little better as my body had had a bit of a break from the chemicals.

"Noooo. Radiation breaks the body down even further. You will find this round *very* tough. Be prepared, Andrea, this one will hit you *hard.*" Dr. Scott had been quite frank in our last meeting. I reminded her that all of my chemos had hit me unusually hard and that it seemed I was a bit of an enigma. She gave me a gentle, awkward smile. I could tell she was concerned. Her eyes said, *Heed my warning, Andrea. I am not trying to scare you, but it will indeed be a challenge.* I had once more travelled to the city to get the requisite blood work and consults coming into Round #5 and was Just. So. Done.

As usual, anxiety hit and I had tears the night before chemo was to begin again. Once more I packed my bag and double-checked all of my meds for the return home—steroids, Gravol, Tylenol, hydromorphone, Claritin. I'd gotten into the habit of packing what I might need if I ended up back in emerge with another long wait. Morning came all too quickly and we headed in. It was August 8, the date of my best friend's birthday. I wished I could have seen her on her special day. I mentally added to my list another special moment I wasn't able to be a part of this year.

My morning update to my online friends was short and simple. A definite sign of my fatigue and defeat.

Social Media Post #14
August 8

Chemo Round #5
That is all.

As a former public school music teacher, I frequently ran into past students. I was often quite pleased to see them, and they often looked overjoyed to see me. I did my best to recall their names; I taught elementary school, and a lot of growth and physical change happens in the years after they move on from that level. Junior high and high school transform them as they find their style and identities. Oftentimes I would still remember a face but not necessarily a name; nevertheless, I would reconnect anyway. I've taught close to four thousand students in several parts of Nova Scotia, so I prided myself any time I correctly recalled someone I'd taught.

During one of my earlier chemo rounds, I recognized one of my former students, now a nurse on the chemo floor; she'd come over to check my beeping machine. She was not my assigned nurse that day but was helping out with a few patients when she noticed she was needed. I looked at her name tag. I remembered I had taught her roughly ten years earlier, when she was just a little kid.

"Emily?" I asked, and she smiled at me. "I taught you elementary music in Sackville!"

She looked at me, bald and not exactly recognizable, in my opinion. "Mrs. Ritcey! I thought that was you! I recognized you the minute you walked in." she replied, excited.

Well. That was impressive. She had identified me after ten years, and I had no hair.

"Well done!" I laughed. We caught up briefly, and I was pleased to see she was doing well.

I very much believe that what goes around, comes around and therefore I live my life in a way that nothing comes back to bite me. I will often say, "Don't burn your bridges, because karma will come for you." I tell my fellow teacher friends that someday their students might become their bosses, so always treat them with kindness and respect. I was glad to have taken my own advice, because I walked in for chemo Round #5 and Emily greeted me even more happily this time—she was assigned as my nurse on this day. After a bit of banter, I teased her and said, "Good thing you liked me all those years back or you could really make today totally miserable!"

She smiled. "I reviewed your file this morning and I know all about your trouble with needles." I was sort of worried, as I didn't want to pass out or have a bad reaction and for Emily to feel like it was her fault. In classic teacher style, I wanted her to have an opportunity to shine.

"Emily, if things go badly today, I want you to know that I believe in you. I know you are smart and that you are *more* than capable." I was worried she would be nervous. "Remember, it's not you, it's me!"

She smiled. "I'm going to give it a go. I think we will be okay."

I'll be darned, the young student was right. She got the needle in me in the very first attempt! I practically cried. I praised her heavily and said how grateful and impressed I was. She looked genuinely pleased. I asked her to call her supervisor over, and I gave her a glowing report on how well Emily did. Once more, it was a very long, nerve-wracking day, but we got through it. I happily left, thinking, *One more chemo and I am DONE!*

Just as Dr. Scott had warned, chemo #5 hit me fast and hard. If this round was a boxing match, I'd say I was the underdog facing a world champ heavyweight and was thrown a hefty haymaker; knocked out in the first round. I had no fight, no energy, and crashed quickly. The drive home was miserable, and I staggered through the doors dizzy, in pain, and very weak. I immediately went to bed.

A few hours later I woke up and began violently vomiting and seeing the all too familiar black tunnels as I stood up. Once more my heart rate soared and my blood pressure plummeted. My temperature rose. I tried my best to drink water, wanting to get the toxins out as best I could. With chemo, some things can taste really "off", and unfortunately for me, one of those off things was water. Our well water had a ton of minerals in it, and even with the filtration system, my body rejected it.

I desperately struggled to get enough fluids in. We tried everything—flat water with lemon, Gatorade, coconut water, sparkling water, and even flavoured drops added to the water. None of it helped. I drank teas and broth but my body reacted a great deal worse with this round. Drinking water and staying properly hydrated was an absolute must in order to flush out both the chemicals and the dying cells. When you can't get them out fast enough, it really does a number on your stomach and I laid in bed, drooling. Ultimately the nausea became too much, and I began forcefully vomiting all over again. This in turn brought on more dehydration and my fever continued to climb. I suffered on and off like this for five days straight. By day six my temperature rose to 102°F. I was supposed to go to Emerge if it was 100. (Dr. Scott had lowered my threshold from 100.4 to 100, and I knew the importance of following this guideline.)

That night as I watched my temperature creep slowly higher, hovering now at 102.3, I made a terrible choice. I took a terrible risk and chose not to go to the hospital. Completely broken, I just couldn't bring myself to face more blood tests, more needles, and I physically could not sit in a waiting room. I knew that. Part of me debated bringing a quilt so I could lie on the floor if need be, but ultimately I reasoned that I was apt to pick up a dangerous superbug off the floor and that it was better that I not go in at all.

Mike came to check on me as I laid there moaning. He was very concerned. "Did you take your temperature?" he asked. I knew if I told him it was over 102 he would have carried me to the car that instant.

"I did, yes," I feebly replied.

"And . . . ?" he asked anxiously.

At that moment, which in hindsight seems horribly awful, I lied.

"It's 99.3. I'm still good."

He didn't look at the thermometer; he *trusted* me. Secretly I was relieved.

That's how very sick I was. I couldn't even deal with a car ride or a waiting room. Ultimately I was told by Dr. Scott that I should have called an ambulance that night, but I just wasn't thinking clearly. I suffered and suffered and suffered all through that night, very afraid but fully accepting that I might actually die. I was just too far gone to do anything about it.

Now that I am through everything, it is clear to me that in this round I had reached the darkest part of my cancer journey, completely ready to give up. In hindsight, I was extremely lucky to have pulled through this round as I was so sick, weak, and completely defeated.

The next morning, I checked my temp again and it had not lessened any through the night. Marginally more rested than the night before, I conceded. "Mike, please take me to emerg." I had no tears left and just stared off into space as he quietly packed my things.

On the drive in, my chest pained so badly, I was concerned again that I might have a heart attack. When we got to emerg they took me in quickly and ran an EKG. At least that was normal. I was taken back out to the waiting room as there were no beds available. The waiting room was heavily crowded, worse than I had ever seen. I sat there in my wheelchair, bald head exposed for all to see, feebly waving my yellow card at the triage nurses and desperately trying to get their attention.

People were crowded all around me as I suffered. I became hugely anxious in my dangerously susceptible, weakened state, knowing that if I were coughed on or touched by someone, I might catch the ever evolving COVID flu or a chest infection, either of which could potentially kill me. I knew I likely once again had very low neutrophils.

I politely asked the two women closest to me to stand back. They were oblivious and chatting away as they stood almost touching me. One of them coughed without covering her mouth. I had had enough. "Move please," I said, my head in my hands, too sick to even hold my head up. They didn't move. "Can you move, please!" I said louder, head still in hands. I was too weak to even look at them. One of them stepped backwards and bumped my wheelchair, jerking it; she was completely clueless. That was my breaking point. "Move!" I bellowed as loudly as I could. It startled them both. They spun around to see me there, crying and furious. "Keep the six-feet-apart rule! Please! I am severely immune-compromised!" I couldn't cope. I started sobbing and was completely embarrassed and flustered.

Mike wheeled me through the crowds to another spot. I waited again in misery as a man in a wheelchair chatted loudly and crudely about a bar fight he had had the night before. He had no respect for anyone feeling sick and needing quiet, and I was floored by his ignorance; he, too, was perfectly clueless about anyone around him. He wheeled up close to me and continued his loud, obnoxious story. I glared at him. Finally, he saw my face and looked confused, probably wondering why I was glaring a death stare at him. I have often wondered why there is not a charge nurse walking around keeping the emergency room quiet and orderly, but alas, it is yet another sign of a very broken system.

With much effort and sheer desperation, I began waving my yellow card like I was a Girl Guide back in the Bedford Troop, with the giant, flowy flag. I got dirty looks from many, who were likely not aware of the protocol and the importance of my yellow card. I finally had a triage nurse come over and say, "You have a yellow card?"

Sheer exasperation for me. "Yes. I told the security check-in person as soon as I arrived."

"Oh. She didn't tell us." She looked at my very short, spiky hair. It had started coming back in during radiation. "I didn't know you had cancer, I just thought you were bald because . . . well, you never can tell these days. Come with me."

Finally, I was taken to the back area behind the triage station and the blood work began again.

35
LEVITICUS

Oh, lovely, I thought as I was finally wheeled to an actual patient room in the emerg. A young man sat at the edge of his bed with his arms feebly wrapped around a barf bucket. *I get to lie here in misery listening to someone puking. Of course.*

I put my head in my hands to shield myself from the scene as Mike wheeled me past. I weakly climbed up into my bed and noticed that the curtain between us and the barfing guy was pretty thin. I could hear him crying and talking. *Who is he talking to?* There was no one with him. Feeling vulnerable, I pondered, *Is he mentally unstable?* I wondered if he might be on the phone, but I didn't think so, he was not speaking loudly enough for anyone on the other end to even hear him.

My nurse came in and attempted to get more blood work done. I explained for the billionth time about my baby-sized veins and that I needed the best "needler" in emerg to do it. She smiled and told me she was pretty confident she could do it, no problem. I looked at my husband. He shrugged at me like, *What can I do?* She began. The tight tourniquet, the vein inspection, and sure enough, the *hmms* ensued.

"Uh, what arm do they usually get the blood out of?" she inquired.

I mumbled, "Whichever arm they can find a vein."

She grumbled a bit and continued to inspect. She turned my arm over and then back again. "Wow, you really *don't* have any good ones, do you?"

She sounded surprised, even though I had literally just explained this to her. She undid the tourniquet and switched arms. All the while, barfing guy was crying and mumbling. Same process on the right arm. "Wow," she said, "these are the tiniest veins I've ever seen!" *Noooo kidding*, I thought. *If only there was a prize for them; I'd take first place.* "Okay, I'm going back to the other arm, I think I saw something better over there."

Five minutes passed as she tap-tap-tapped on my left arm.

"Would it help you if I sat up and hung my arm down?" I asked. "Gravity can make my blood expand the veins in my hand." I was starting to dread what I knew was inevitably going to happen.

"No, no, I'm good. I think I found one." There was the familiar smell of rubbing alcohol as she wiped the spot. Then she said, "Okay, this is just going to sting a wee bit." And she was absolutely right that it stung, but it stung a lot more than a wee bit. And again that familiar moving around as she dug into my vein as it rolled. She held her breath and winced. "I'm really sorry," she said through a screwed-up face.

"It's okay." I clenched my teeth and my toes. And then, agonizing pain.

"Oh gosh, I blew right through your vein. I am so sorry."

She undid the tourniquet, removed the needle and put the usual cotton ball and tape over me. She smiled apologetically and came around to the other arm again. "Okay." She sounded determined. "I think I can get it this time." She took even longer looking, tapping, turning and finally decided to go ahead on her mission.

"Ow!" I yelled, making her jump.

"Oh shoot! I am SO sorry!" She burst through another vein as I tried not to cry. It really hurts when this happens, my veins are just so beat up. I took another deep breath. She stood up. "I'm going to go get Allen, our paramedic. He's really, *really* good at this!" She hurriedly left and buddy next to me continued to quietly moan.

After a while, a tall, friendly man came in, all smiles and confidence. "Well, hello there!" he said.

"Ah! You must be Allen." I smiled, weakly. I beat him to the punch.

"They tell me you're causing some trouble in here," he said calmly.

"Yup. That's me." It's the usual banter before the torture, but my usual upbeat voice is flat, depressed, defeated.

"Okay," Allen said, "I gotta warn ya, you're not going to like me very much, but I *will* get this done."

Oh God, give me strength.

He inspected my arms. Both of them. For quite a while. "I will only poke when I am one hundred percent certain, okay?"

He decided upon the veins in the inner part of my wrist; a delicate, tender spot. Out came the rubbing alcohol for the wipe-down. He actually hummed while he got ready.

"Okay, do you want a countdown?" He smiled.

"Nope," I said, ready to have a heart attack. "Just do it."

He carefully and slowly inserted the needle. "Oh my God, I am so sorry," he said as he placed it in one of the tiniest veins of my inner wrist. "But, I got it in."

"What?" I cried in disbelief. "You did? Oh my gosh, Allen, thank you, thank you, thank you! I love you sooo much!"

He chuckled, happy for the feedback. "Don't love me yet; we still gotta fill these five bottles of blood!"

Now, you may be thinking these are the usual little vials they use, but no. These were actually much larger bottles with other liquids in them as well that they send off for blood cultures. Sooo much blood to be taken from sooo little a vein.

"Let's get these done and see how things go!" he said.

I laid there, listening to each bottle get opened and closed. I was silently praying. *Don't break the vein, don't let the blood flow stop, don't break the vein, don't let the blood flow stop.*

"Okay! All done now, Andrea!"

Big relief. HUGE. "Can I clone you?" I begged.

He laughed and put his hand on my arm. "No, you may not. But do please ask for me whenever you are here. If I am working, I will come help you."

He left just as quickly as he had appeared. Greatly relieved, yet sick and feverish, I was all smiles again, even with the stinging pulse in my left wrist.

The nurse came back and started getting the bottles ready for the lab, and then I heard my husband say, "Uh, your buddy tipped over." The nurse swiftly moved past us and to the other patient. I could overhear them and learned that he was on Valium and they were trying to sort him out.

Before long, a doctor from the oncology team came in the room. By this point, I felt so poorly, I could barely keep my eyes open. I was in a great deal of pain. She carefully inspected my tummy and found the same very painful spot that had plagued me for months, ever since my surgery. She pushed on it and I yelped. She didn't know if it was an abscess or what.

"We are going to get a CT scan and a chest X-ray for starters," she said. They wanted to rule out clots and heart attacks. "First I will get you something for your pain. Can you take morphine?" she asked.

"Yes." I replied, and then fell asleep in exhaustion.

I woke up to a voice saying, "Okay, Andrea, this might feel a little funny, but try to ride the wave, okay?" In went 5 mg of liquid morphine. It hit me instantly and I felt a little anxious with the immediate high. *This must be similar to what heroin feels like.* I was flying high.

"Whoa, I feel reeeally weeeird . . ." I could hear myself talking but it was as if I was hearing someone else from outside my head. My voice sounded like I was the ultimate stoner. I began to panic. Mike was by my side and someone was rubbing my forehead. There were hands on my arms. "You're okay, just ride the wave. It'll pass in a minute."

"Whoa, this is sooo trippyyy. I feel so high . . ."

I promptly fall asleep.

When I woke up, I had to pee. Garbage bucket buddy was still next to me and still crying and whispering. The nurse told me there was a bathroom down the hall. I explained that I was waaaay toooooo hiiiigh to get there and asked if there was a toilet in the little cupboard that I could use. My husband looked at me like I was nuts.

"There sure is!" the nurse said, and she pulled open the cupboard door to show a little toilet. So amazing. She handed me a white plastic hat and I slowly sat up.

"Do you want me to leave to give you some privacy?" buddy next to us asked. *My gosh*, I thought to myself, *he's so thoughtful, even in his terribly ill state.*

"No, hunny," I said. "I'm okay. If you don't care, I don't care." I mean honestly, after you have a baby and the whole world has seen you with your legs pinned over your head, does anything ever really matter after that?

I got up carefully and slowly. I got the job done and climbed back into bed. Hubby left to go use a real bathroom. Now it was just buddy and me alone in the room for the first time. A few minutes pass. I still hear him crying. It's killing me. I want to help.

"Are you okay, sweetie?" I ask

"No." He sounds so devastated.

"Can I help at all?"

And he jumped right in, both feet. "I'm an alcoholic. My girlfriend is about to leave me. I can't lose her. I just can't. She's all I've got. She lost a baby a few months ago. We're so devastated . . . . I can't seem to stop drinking."

Holy moly. I was not expecting him to open up like that. My heart instantly went out to him. I wanted to get up and give him a hug.

We ended up talking for hours. Mike had returned to our full-on, heavy conversation, and he quietly put his head into his computer as buddy and I talked and talked and talked. We shared a tremendous amount of stuff. I suggested numerous ideas to help him overcome his addiction. I was so very touched by how forthcoming and honest he was.

He asked me a lot about myself and I shared my journey and how much I was struggling but yet how close I was getting to the finish line. A boxing theme of my journey solidified when he randomly said, "You didn't fight this hard only to die in the last round." I thought about that, long and hard. He was absolutely right. It gave me exactly the fighting edge I needed to finish my "opponent" off.

The time came for buddy to be discharged. I overheard him tell the nurse he was going to walk home. I couldn't see him past the curtains, but I was very worried for him. He started to say thank you for the talk and the ear and I said, "Do you want to exchange info? I really care about your well-being and want to help you if I can."

He sounded like he was in disbelief as he stammered, "Y-yes . . . yes; I would like that . . . very much." I could tell he was smiling as we exchanged numbers. "What is your name?" I asked gently. "Leviticus," he said, and quietly left.

He and I became fast friends, and he credits me regularly for saving his life. To this day, he and I check in every few days, and he has remained sober, maintaining and excelling in his job and doing great. He is in full recovery. He has a lot to offer in humour, uniqueness, and love, and I am grateful that we met.

An elderly man came into the room, all smiles. "Hello, young lady!" he said to me. "I've come to take you away. Are you wearing a bra?"

Now *this* got my attention. He was about eighty. His name tag said "Parker." I cracked up laughing and said, "Well, Parker, I am in fact *not* wearing a bra. I bet it's not every day that you come up to a woman and ask her that!"

Without missing a beat, he replied, "Well actually, it's not every day that I have to help them take it *off*!"

He went on to explain that you can't have a bra on for a chest X-ray. The metal wires and clips mess everything up. So off we went for X-rays. I was still super high from the morphine. I couldn't stand for the X-ray pictures, so they propped me up with huge triangular pillows and got it all sorted out. Parker swiftly wheeled me back, and I forced myself to refrain from apologizing for the big workout he was likely having, pushing the heavy bed with me in it.

Not long after the chest X-ray they took me down for the CT scan. A friendly man with very curly grey hair introduced himself while I was in the hall waiting for my turn in the scan. He picked up my arm and instantly cringed. "Oh my God, what have they done to you?" His face was all twisted.

"What, the IV?"

"Yeah," he says. "I hate seeing them there. That's such a tender spot."

I explained my situation as he observed the two burst vein spots on my middle arms that were already bruising past the Band-Aids.

"Oh, you poor thing." He sighed deeply.

"Is this CT scan with dye?" I nervously inquired.

"Yes, hun, it is. Would you like me to try and get a better IV set up?"

I almost jumped out of the bed and ran down the hall. "No, this was the best they could do. They had to get a paramedic named Allen to do this."

His eyebrows shot up. "This is *Allen's* work?"

"Yes." I sniffed.

He sighed. "Oh boy, you *must* have bad veins . . . ."

In I went for the CT scan. The technician introduced herself and I showed her my IV site. "Oh, Andrea. I'm not gonna lie, this is going to hurt."

"I know," I replied in defeat. *When will this freaking end?*

"When I do the saline and dye, I'm going to do it as slowly as I can, okay? You let me know if it gets to be too much."

The machines moved me into the gigantic grey doughnut as I counted in my head how many scans I was at now. I think for a minute, in my still feverish state. One for the hysterectomy. One in February to check my pain issues while still admitted. One in April after chemo Round #1. One in June after chemo Round #3. Two in late June getting ready for radiation. And one now. I think there was one other, but I've lost count.

I put my arms over my head and try to get comfortable as the IV tubes tug slightly. It's super uncomfortable holding my arms in this position, and my back begins cramping. The machine shoots the saline in. I jump and yell, "Ow!" quite loudly. It startles them, and I quickly call again, "I'm sorry!" I need to wear a sign on my forehead warning the staff that I am an abrupt yeller as my veins are in such bad shape.

I begin the scans with my eyes tightly closed. This helps me not feel claustrophobic. It always helps to close your eyes *before* the machine brings you into the doughnut hole, so you don't see what a tight fit it is all around you. I wished I didn't have to hear the noisy machine though, as you really cannot stick your fingers in your ears.

"Okay, Andrea, here we go with the dye." I felt her put her hand over my wrist and slightly press down on the IV area. I think this protected me from the pain somewhat and slowed down the process even further to avoid a gush of liquid blowing up my vein. It helped, but it still hurt immensely. I sucked in air and clenched my whole body—a great butt workout.

"Just breathe if you can," I heard. Her hand was so comforting. *Dear Lord, please get this done.* It really was stinging now.

Finally it was finished and she said, "Okay, just another shot of saline and you're good to go." Another shot indeed. It squirts in from a machine and the gauge is clearly bigger than my veins.

"Ow!" I yell loudly again, followed by another "Sorry!"

They wheel me back into my emerg room and another couple is in there now; the man is having a heart attack. Before too long, my doc comes in and tells me they don't like that my neutrophils are super low and that they are going to start me on a very powerful drug as they don't want to wait any longer. They are worried about sepsis. I become even more anxious at the thought of an antibiotic as I am allergic to almost every one and I don't know how I will react to this. I am told we don't really have a choice, but they are all geared up if I have another anaphylactic reaction like I did in chemo Round #2.

"Okay," I said, "go for it."

She injects the medicine. After a few minutes, when I realize I am not going to die, I fall asleep.

The duty doc returns and tells me I am being admitted again to the VG. She explains that it will take several hours for an ambulance to become available for transport and that it would be better if Mike just takes me. They carefully wrap up my IV site in clean white cotton bandaging so that the IV doesn't snag or pull out, and off we go. This time we decide to drive to McDonald's first before we land at the next hospital. I mean a girl's gotta eat, right?

36

THE HOSPITAL IS NO PLACE FOR THE SICK

Hospital Stay #3

Again, I arrived to the Victoria General Hospital. To my surprise, they actually remembered me from a few months ago, and I was wheeled to a room shared with one other woman. It was not long before I realized she was a patient living with dementia. She kept talking to me and saying things that I carefully answered so that I didn't confuse her further.

Two young nurses came in. They looked at my IV site, which had become red and puffy, and they told me they had to remove it and give me a new one. I burst into tears and refused. I politely explained that it felt fine and that Allen the paramedic did it. I described all that I had been through with ruptured veins, the vast issues getting the needles in, the pain I'd endured while they made their attempts, and how I had zero coping skills left. They left, quietly talking.

After a few minutes they came back, looking very empathetic, and said, "We are so very sorry, but your IV does not look safe and it can get infected. You need a new one to withstand all the medications we have to give you." This thought absolutely terrified me as my body was just so tired. Still high on morphine, you would think I wouldn't have minded, but I very much did. "We could give you an Ativan if that helps?" one of the young nurses offered. *That might work . . . I would still feel the pain but not as much from the morphine, and the Ativan would take away my terror, or, at least, lessen it . . .* At this point I would take an anti-anxiety drug ANY DAY. I came to terms with the offer, thinking that this might actually be an okay solution.

"Yes, okay, I will try. But please, if you can, do it really carefully, I still don't want to be a pin cushion!" I smiled at them as best I could, desperately trying not to come off as *that* patient. They left again.

Back in a flash, they gave me the Ativan, and thirty minutes later I was feeling moderately okay about the idea of another IV attempt.

"I'm going to use a baby size gauge that we use in neo-natal," one of them said. This actually sounded promising for my tiny veins. And, miracle of miracles, she got it in.

She told me I needed potassium, and I emphatically explained through gritted teeth, "I will jump out this window right now if you even come near me with a potassium bag—I swear this on my life." She looked at me with such pity, there was no doubt she could tell I was serious. Not wanting to make enemies in the hospital, I backed off a bit and added, "Sorry, ladies. It's been a long haul and I *legitimately* have zero coping skills." They immediately brought in a potassium pill; I swallowed it happily and promptly fell asleep.

I woke up in the dark, roughly an hour later, to clonky, heavy footsteps. I opened my eyes to see a strange, toothless man smiling at me from behind a curtain.

"Yes?" I said, in a commanding, strong voice. He had startled me and I felt scared but didn't let on. "Can I help you?" I asked again, my heart pounding. He stared for a full minute longer as I started to get really creeped out.

"Where's my bed?" he asked in a confused state.

I quickly replied, "Not here!"

He backed up and stopped. I heard him breathing heavily and waiting for several minutes just on the other side of the curtain. He shuffled a few steps, and then the bed next to me creaked; I assume he had laid down. He was there for several more minutes and then a nurse came and told him he was in the wrong room. *What is going on here?* I was surrounded by dementia patients and wondered if I was in fact on the cancer floor or somewhere else.

Two hours later they woke me up and moved me to a private room. It was the very same room I had stayed in the last time I was admitted, and I was greatly relieved to be in a single. I asked how I was so lucky to get my own room, and they explained that this was the floor for the overflow of dementia patients and that I certainly did not need to be dealing with that after all I'd been through. I decided to alert my online family that I had again been admitted.

Social Media Post #15
August 16

Hey peeps!
I've been admitted back into the VG.
I'll be fine, but wanted to try and combat all the texts.

Satisfied and exhausted, I gratefully fell into a deep, although fitful, sleep. I hoped I would not have any more weird narcotic dreams like the water sorceress who still haunted me on occasion. I slept off and on until the wee hours of the morning, and then the business of the hospital began.

6:00 a.m.   I startle awake as a strange man quietly enters my room. Without a word, he places a cup of water on my bed tray and exits, equally as silent.

6:45 a.m.   I hear the next shift of nurses gathering in the hall. My room is right across from the front desk where the new staff gather and the worn-out staff finish. It is a great party as they all congregate and greet each other and encourage each other. They have no concept of the noise they make, but it is a happy group of voices so I don't mind—just impossible to sleep, so I wait till they dissipate.

7:00 a.m.   I drift off and startle awake again to see another man has quietly entered and is now towering over me, getting ready to take my blood. It is extremely painful as my blood does not want to come out.

7:30 a.m.   Just as I settle from the blood draw, a third man enters, dropping off a breakfast tray. I eat rubbery eggs and dry toast, hurriedly, as I plan to catch a nap after I finish.

8:00 a.m.   A nurse appears, does a vitals check (body temperature, respiration rate, oxygen levels, pulse rate, blood pressure). She listens to my chest and then hooks up my IV for a forty-five-minute antibiotic and saline drip. All looks good. She stays talking with me for a number of minutes as I yawn and flutter my eyelids. She doesn't notice.

8:45 a.m.   I attempt to sleep.

9:00 a.m.   The oncology doctor arrives to check on me, and afterward, I attempt again to sleep.

10:00 a.m.   A cleaning lady comes in and mops the floor, empties garbage cans, loudly snaps new bags in place, and sings wholeheartedly as she works. She leaves and I drift off.

11:00 a.m.   The pharmacy guy arrives, wakes me up, and wants to review all my meds. We chat for about twenty minutes and then I attempt yet again to doze off.

12:00 p.m.   Nurse #1 enters for another vitals check. Yay, all normal. She chats about how she used to live in Alberta and misses milking her cows . . .

1:00 p.m.   A fourth unfamiliar man appears with my lunch tray—a grilled cheese sandwich and Jell-O.

2:00 p.m.   Nurse #1 arrives for my second IV hookup for the forty-five-minute antibiotic and saline drip, chats away, and fiddles with the machine as it keeps beeping at her. She doesn't talk about cows but rather how she has ADHD and doesn't think her meds are working.

2:55 p.m.   I attempt to doze off.

3:00 p.m.   Man #3 returns to take my lunch tray and wants to discuss the dinner selection. We review the list of six choices and end up talking about my food allergies.

4:00 p.m.   A new nurse arrives for vitals check #3. My temp and blood pressure are up, as well as my heart rate. No surprise there. I drift off.

5:00 p.m.   I startle awake as man #4 enters for dinner tray drop-off. It's not what I ordered, but I eat it anyway, thinking someone else just got my pizza. I stay awake and do a Sudoku puzzle. Then I do five more.

6:00 p.m.   Man #4 collects my dinner tray and I tell him my dinner got mixed up. He smiles and says, "Very good-good-good," and walks out. He speaks very little English. I doze off.

6:45 p.m.   The nurses' party starts up again. I hear robust singing of "Happy Birthday," then some clapping, some big announcement, etc. It is delightful to hear how close they all are and how spirited they feel, yet also, mildly annoying.

7:00 p.m.	Sleeeeeep. Please. Let me just sleeeeeep.
8:00 p.m.	Nurse #2 is back for vitals check #4 and decides to get me some Tylenol as my temp is up. She hooks my IV back up for my third round of the forty-five-minute antibiotic and saline drip and tells me there are some Alzheimer's patients on our floor, but they are very quiet except this one man, Mr. Dong, who is friendly but acts up at night. I try not to think or worry about what that means. I explain how tired I am. I am told there is nothing more scheduled for me and that I can probably get some sleep. I check my watch; it is 8:55 p.m. I get all snuggly and attempt some sleep.
9:00 p.m.	I awaken to horribly loud pounding and a man yelling, "Let me out! Let. Me. Out!" I hear the nurses trying to redirect and distract him. They coax him to go for a walk. The banging and yelling continues. Then I hear in a panicked voice, "Mr. Dong, put the chair down. Put the chair down, Mr. Dong, right now. Don't throw that chair!" and then a loud smashing of glass. Then I hear on the intercom, "Code 5, Code White, Code 5, Code White. I repeat—Code 5, Code White, Code 5, Code White." I lie there in my bed feeling scared and vulnerable as this is just outside my door. Ultimately security comes and locks him in his room. He continues to yell off and on for two more hours.
10:00 p.m.	I settle. And then my phone starts blowing up with check-ins and messages, and I have to finally turn on the "Do not disturb." Close to eleven o'clock I doze off.
11:00 p.m.	I wake up just as New Nurse #3 stabs me with a blood thinner spring-press pokey thing in my leg that leaves a lump.

Apparently when you "laze around all day in bed" you can develop blood clots.

12:00 a.m.   I fall asleep briefly and then nurse #3 wakes me for vitals check #5. Temp is better. Heart rate and blood pressure are up. I try and sleep.

1:00 a.m.   Oh. My. God. I can't sleep.

2:00 a.m.   Nurse #3 hooks my IV up for yet another forty-five-minute antibiotic and saline drip. Is this Round #4 today? I . . . think . . . so.

3:00 a.m.   ZZZZZZZzzzzzzzZZZZZZZzzzzzzzZZZZZZZzzzzzzz

4:00 a.m.   Woken up for vitals check #6. Just let me die already. I drift off.

5:00 a.m.   OMG, I wake up again. I'm soaking wet with hot flashes and itchy legs and pain in my back. I settle and drift off.

6:00 a.m.   I startle awake as a strange man quietly enters my room. Without a word, he places a cup of water on my bed tray and exits, equally as silent.

This hamster wheel continues for the entire week that I am there. I am desperate to get off.

The staff were amazed that my teeny little vein held on for dear life and that the teeny neo-natal IV gauge steadfastly soldiered on. The very painful blood draws during this hospital stay totalled nine. As I write this, countless months later, I still have bruising on the insides of both forearms. Perhaps permanent damage from nine more blood draws, five press needles of blood thinners, and the several IV attempts in emerg that last fateful night. My arms are a mess. To my surprise, I also ended up with painful lumps deep under my skin from each blood thinner injection.

Several of my friends and family members came in to visit during my weeklong admission. Mike was in for a few minutes almost every day, Annie and Maddie came a few times with beautiful flowers, my parents both saw me. Marianne popped in, bringing me a delicious coffee and snack; she had driven all over the city to find my favourite coffee. Sue cooked my favourite dinner, Greek lemon chicken. She brought it in with a yummy side, and the dish came complete with a knife and fork and a wee napkin. We hung out and I shared with her that I was thinking about writing a book about this whole awful cancer journey.

One day, one of my very astute guitar friends, Jane, checked in with me. I briefly shared what I was dealing with, trying so hard to be positive even though I was so greatly discouraged. She saw right through it and said, "Andrea, none of us will ever know how much courage you have had to tap into Every. Single. Day." I was brought to tears by her insightful acknowledgement. It was so accurate. Only the cancer patients and their partners know the nitty-gritty of the twenty-four-hours-a-day experiences; the heavy, raw emotions; and the bravery we have to have on a daily, sometimes hourly, sometimes moment-to-moment basis. Generally, the outside world knows very little about all that's entailed in this long battle to survive. I completely understand now why, sadly, some warriors give up.

During my stay, my mind repeatedly fretted over the fact that I was now overdue to start using the vaginal dilator to protect from stenosis. The staff repeatedly said, "You're okay. Don't you worry about that." In hindsight, I should not have trusted that they knew anything about my situation. I really should have "worried" about it, got Mike to bring the thing in—anything to help prevent future issues. But I was so sick, mildly constipated again from being in the hospital, and still dealing with large, painful, external hemorrhoids, I don't think I would have been able to use the darn thing anyway.

I had been in hospital for a week, with no sleep and far too many needles, meds, blood tests, and yucky meals. Late afternoon on day six, I still didn't know when I would be discharged. Every day, my neutrophils continued to remain low. "Weird," a nurse said. "They should be on their way back up by now . . . ." I worried that I would feel weak for months on end and started to feel even gloomier. Each morning they poked me and drew blood, and by mid-morning I knew my fate was another day in jail.

The morning of day seven, Dr. Scott came in and we had a long talk about my last several months and how brutally awful it had been up to this point.

"How are you feeling about doing your last chemo?" She looked at me with concern, knowing how miserable I was.

I looked at her, trying to find the words. I didn't want to sound overly dramatic; my answer was a watered down version of my intense feelings. "Quite frankly, I'm ready to jump off the nearest bridge."

She knew it. She told me she felt that I had been through enough, and that if I felt like it, I could be done.

Done! Well! My thoughts raced. Although I felt enormous relief, interestingly my first thought was, *But I'll never get to ring the bell!* I was surprised at how strong my feelings were about that. Out of months and months of working so hard and trying to stick with the treatments and hating every minute of them, the thought of a big, giant party and ringing the bell with absolute fervour at the cancer centre was what was getting me through. It was the light at the end of the tunnel, an official mark that I was indeed finished treatment. It showed that I was tough enough to get through them all. It provided a sense of accomplishment, and it was the beginning of time to celebrate. *Not* ringing the bell felt, dare I say, anticlimactic.

I tried my hardest to control my conflicting emotions. Then the realization that she was saying I could truly be done actually dawned on me. The enormous relief, the immense gratitude, the let-down of adrenalin and nerves and worry all hit me at once, and I burst into great, body-wracking sobs, as if I had been holding my breath for months.

Dr. Scott instantly realized just how much I had been holding back and looked at me with much empathy. We had a mutual appreciation for one another; it had been hard for her to see me struggle so much. It must get to be all too much for the oncologist at times like these; I can only imagine the misery they see.

After a few more minutes of blowing my nose and shaking with emotion, I started to settle.

"I think you like the idea then?" She smiled.

I did indeed, yes.

"Well, let's see where you're at in your next checkup after they release you, and we can decide then, okay?"

Even though I wanted to be finished more than anything, I still thought about standard treatment protocol. I struggled a bit making the decision to be finished because I truly did worry that I might become sick again. I began researching the stats and found there is not much research available regarding the pros and cons of stopping at five vs. six rounds, although six is the suggested ideal number overall.

Quite honestly, though, at this point, I really *did* fear that I would not make it through Round #6—either the infusion would kill me, the aftermath of pain, weakness, and the dangerously low neutrophils and electrolytes might, or I might somehow be exposed in the hospital to COVID or another powerful bug and have nothing left to fight it off. Heck, even if I physically got through, the mental anguish and suffering might do me in. I felt that if I had to cope with one more of even the tiniest of things, I would indeed look for the nearest bridge, ledge, or window. My resources to draw from had completely, truly vanished, and my PTSD was at an all-time high. My body had fought the fight and I was beyond done. I knew, indisputably, I was done-done.

37
STENOSIS

On the morning of day eight they told me I was safe enough to go home. Even though my neutrophils were still alarmingly low (I was reading 0.2 and ideally should be at 4), I was at least out of the extreme danger zone of infection, having been on powerful antibiotics for eight days. I was instructed to continue the antibiotics at home for another week. I know Dr. Scott preferred for me to remain in hospital even a few days longer, but I strongly suspected they needed the bed. I was still in very rough shape when I was discharged, but I was more than ready to go home and to just be completely finished with everything.

Social Media Post #16
August 23

Hey Peeps! I'm released from hospital. Yay!!!!
My neutrophils are at 0.2 so I am again living in isolation, but at least I'm out!!

Even after I was released, I continued to be plagued by fevers, abdominal pain, and enormous, tender, external hemorrhoids that lasted at least another month. I was still suffering the repercussions of that damned seven-pound clay baby back in April and then further irritated by the radiation effects.

I started to think about the road to recovery and was really missing having a normal relationship with my husband. I missed our friendship, our partying, and most of all, our intimacy. A year of issues, severe bleeding, and pain before the cancer diagnosis followed by the miserable ten months with the hysterectomy, the chemo, the radiation, and three hospital stays post cancer diagnosis—intimacy with Mike was pretty low on our list.

I wanted to plan a trip somewhere when this nightmare was all over, to recover physically but more importantly, mentally. I needed a major reset, a decompression from all of the trauma that I (we) had endured. Mike needed a big break from all of his extra duties and the sheer stress of watching me suffer. We decided we would go to Naples, Florida. We had gotten engaged there, returned to celebrate our honeymoon and had taken Annie and Maddie twice when they were younger. It was indeed a very special place for us. We booked a trip for the end of October as I didn't want to be at home on the one-year anniversary of my cancer diagnosis, which was coming up quickly. I certainly didn't want to find myself replaying that miserable day in my mind, and I figured being in the warm sunshine in our favourite place would serve us both well.

And so, I focused my efforts on recovery. The multiple, severe health issues pushed me into six weeks' post-radiation before I was able to actually use the vaginal dilator. One day while in the shower, I nervously did just that; and it seemed like everything was all good. *Weird,* I thought, *this seems pretty uneventful, even with being four weeks late to the game.* So a few days later, I quickly checked again, and things seemed okay. I continued on this way for several weeks, not even knowing that the effects of radiation can last up to a year. One day, I felt resistance and pain. *What on earth? Has my bladder dropped?* I was told that the bladder and bowels would shift from the hysterectomy. All of this was very new to me, of course; it was basically a "learn as you go" type of thing.

I dried off from the shower and anxiously went over to the bed. I laid horizontally to try a different position in hopes that the resistance was indeed only my bladder and that it would shift without gravity pulling it down. To my dismay, there was still resistance and pain, and terrifyingly, the months of worry about the potential horrifying condition of stenosis were now, very much, confirmed.

Cringing yet? It's okay—I was too at first. But you know, the parts of the body that have historically been viewed as "private" have always had very complicated things going on with them. In times like these, it is all too necessary to share information and to learn as much as we can about our bodies for our own health and safety, especially as women. I spent countless hours researching and anxiously wondering what was happening to my body without having anyone readily available to ask or with whom to discuss things. It was a very troubling time as I realized that there is very little literature on this subject.

I felt awkward and embarrassed as I searched for information, and then I realized that we all know that inevitably our bodies go through many physical changes from infancy to puberty, sexuality to functionality, procreation to childbirth, and all the health concerns in between, so why *do* we have to be uncomfortable discussing it? Well, it's plain and simple folks —we don't. Let's just decide *not* to be uncomfortable about any of our concerns.

Florida, in my mind, was about reconnecting with Mike in all aspects of our marriage. With the beginnings of stenosis, I was now completely panicked and scrambling to figure out what to do with this very real, very upsetting issue only a few weeks before our trip. I started making calls to pelvic physios and found one who came highly recommended. I began extremely painful appointments, and I was told I had a lot of work to do. The dilator kit comes with five different sizes to choose from based on the severity of the stenosis, and the largest one was still not ergonomically designed like a life-like "member." Instead, it was abnormally narrow at the end and nerve-wrackingly pointy, designed to break through scar tissue. With the shrinking effects of pelvic radiation and brachytherapy, the scarring from being internally fried, the hysterectomy itself, the destruction of my rectum from the seven-pound clay baby and the giant hemorrhoids that followed as well as the damage from chemo, I was basically destroyed inside and out. The pelvic specialist shocked me one day; she felt so much scarring and damage, she couldn't tell what she was feeling. "Do you have mesh or maybe some kind of metal inside here?" she asked, rather harshly. I was horrified to learn that it felt like that.

Scar tissue needs to be broken down (which is quite painful and upsetting), so I met with her a few times a week. I was troubled to learn that I was supposed to do the dilator work for twenty minutes at a time. If only I had been better informed. I am sharing this because people's lives have been destroyed by vaginal stenosis; some have spent years in agony with stenosis affecting the use of menstrual products, painful doctor check-ups, and of course, intimacy. I was certainly not hitting that twenty-minute mark and often wonder how much further ahead I'd have been had I known that from the beginning.

I also learned that things not only can shrink in length but also in width. The vaginal wall muscles can get as hard as a rock and become completely inflexible. Surprisingly, this is quite common.

Pelvic health knowledge is extremely important! Through my research I learned you can develop vaginal stenosis from a hysterectomy, from chemotherapy, and of course, more obviously, from pelvic radiation. I want women (and partners) to know about my experience so they can avoid a similar nightmare. I have a long way to go in recovery and am extremely grateful that I have an understanding, patient, and gentle husband in this hellish journey.

To compound the stress and worry of dealing with problems in my nether regions, my hair began to fall out all over again. Losing my hair during my very first round of chemo was awful. The only thing worse than losing your hair to chemo? —losing all of it to chemo . . . *twice!*

My hair had grown in beautifully during the long weeks of radiation, during the "chemo reprieve." It had come in so thick it felt like a rug up top. It was still only a centimetre long at the time, mind you, but it was abundant and full, no bald spots and no chicken fuzz. Each day my hands had habitually gone up to rub my new, soft, thick hair, and I loved the feel of it. It was a relief knowing that it was coming in properly, and I was getting my self-confidence back. I'd heard horror stories of women having issues where their hair came in very slowly, in patches, or never grew at all!

And so, sixteen days after chemo Round #5, all of my newly grown hair began to fall out for the second time. I was emotional and vulnerable and self-conscious and back to my pale, shiny head with little white spriggy bits. When I sat in front of a lamp in the evening, the glow from the light accentuated my spriggy bits and I looked like a baby chicken. I was hugely discouraged. I had known that I was going to go through this a second time, but what I was not prepared for was that it felt even *more* depressing than the first time.

One night I was working hard at trying to feel like my old self. I was discouraged about my bald head, missing the beautiful mane I'd had just over half a year ago. Standing in front of the mirror, my eyes slowly surveyed my body. *Who is this person before me?* My skin was completely dried out from head to toe and looked like it belonged to a weathered old dragon. The five scars from my hysterectomy were still bright red, shiny, and sore. My muscles had completely disappeared, and I took in the now completely Jell-O-like flab all over my arms, my torso, my legs, and I felt the soreness and deep aches from the pains in my pelvic region. My butt was still aching, and each time I peed it burned like I was emptying out broken bits of glass. My chest pained from the heartache of it all, and my spirit was completely, *irrevocably,* broken. I took a breath in and felt my heart pumping faster and faster. My head felt light, like I was floating. My fingers started tingling, and I quickly realized I was starting to have an anxiety attack. I felt angry all of the sudden. Rage-like even. I still didn't understand why this was all happening to me, and I hated the universe for giving me this horrible load to deal with.

I clenched my fists and tried hard to regain control. I knew Mike was out walking Duey, and all of a sudden, a violent urge to scream filled my body. Still standing in front of the mirror, I saw my face turn red and I opened my mouth and I screamed a long, loud, powerful, guttural scream. Breathless, I leaned hard against the wall near me. It felt good to scream. I tilted my head back and screamed hard again and again and again. My throat started to hurt and I began crying. Big fat tears rolled down my cheeks and into my mouth. *When will this nightmare end?* I looked at myself, standing there, now shaking with fury. "I want my body back," I whispered to the girl in the mirror. "I want my hair back," I implored, a little louder. And then those angry feelings hit me even harder and I screamed like an absolute mad woman, "I want my life back! I want my life back! I! Want! My! Life! Baaaack!!"

I fell to the floor in giant, wailing sobs and wished for the thousandth time that this fate was not mine.

PART THREE

🔔🔔🔔

38

THE BEGINNING
OF THE END

Chemo Round #6 was quickly approaching and I knew I had a major decision to make. Dr. Scott's suggestion to be finished after Round #5 weighed heavily on me. I knew of course, that it was best to complete all six rounds and I was deathly afraid the cancer would come back with a vengeance if I skipped the final treatment. However, there was just one teeny problem. I'd been so horribly ill from Round #5, that I was even *more* afraid that going through with the last round might *actually* kill me.

Making the decision felt like I was playing Russian roulette. I desperately wanted to ring the bell; I wanted to complete the protocol. I felt like I'd have bragging rights and feel really proud that I'd "toughed it out" but yet, from the deepest parts of my being, I knew I just couldn't do it.

I went back and forth on this for hours. *How does one make a decision in this situation?* I had the required pre-chemo blood work done and hoped the result would provide some direction. It didn't.

I met with the oncology team and hoped Dr. Scott could help me make the final decision. I was disappointed to see it was a different doctor scheduled that day, although one who was still on the same clinical team. It was normal to get passed around of course, as Dr. Scott was also a surgeon and couldn't always meet with me. Thankfully, this new doctor was also seasoned and kind.

He introduced himself as he came in and I could see by his face that he was very special. He placed his hand on my arm and said, "Andrea. I have spent considerable time reviewing your very large file. You have been through an *extraordinary* amount. How are you feeling?"

My eyes welled up and I tried my hardest not to have yet another darn tear roll down my chemo-puffy face. I knew I'd been through a lot, but hearing the oncologist say this when they deal with patients going through cancer every day, validated that I indeed had gone through a horrific battle. I thought for a moment, trying to articulate how I truly felt. I readied myself and said, "I am well beyond my ability to cope with anything more." My body involuntarily inhaled a quick, shallow breath, and I had to press my tongue hard up behind my front teeth to keep from bursting into full-fledged tears.

He looked at me lying on the examination table, obviously struggling. He considered my reply for a few seconds and nodded contemplatively. We discussed numbers of chemo rounds and their prognosis, my allergic reactions, my hospital admissions and my quality of life . . . or lack thereof. He carefully listened to my opinion on all of those things. And, after a long, thoughtful pause, he said, "In my opinion, I think you are okay to be finished with the chemo. I second Dr. Scott's proposal. Would you like that?"

Oh my god, would I ever.

I just about leapt off the table into his arms shouting, "Yes! Yes! Yeeesssssss!" but I was so overwhelmed in that very moment that I just needed a minute. It was all too much. I laid there on the patient table and simply cried and nodded, lips trembling too much to even speak. I knew if I opened my mouth I would lose all emotional control as it was a gut wrenching, nerve wracking decision.

He smiled. "Very good. I think that's a wrap!"

He quietly left the room and Mike and I looked at each other in disbelief. *We're done? This nightmare is finally over?* Mike stood up and came to me. We held each other in a huge, long embrace. We did it! We got through this terrible, horrific nightmare, barely hanging to the last little fragment of a very worn thread for far too many months. We looked at each other with such tremendous joy and relief—I'll never forget that moment in the Cancer Centre for as long as I live.

"I'll get the car," Mike said. We were ready to go home.

Social Media Post #17
August 28

Sometimes the best laid plans go awry.

6 rounds just got changed to 5.

I'm DONE chemo!!!!

Slowly, I began healing. And in the days following that appointment, I spent a great deal of thought reflecting back on the past year. Dealing with the cancer diagnosis, the surgery, chemo, radiation, debilitating damage, and the long road to recovery, I realized that the physical and emotional aftermath of this disease is long, hard going and messy. Painfully, I also realized that there's a *social* aftermath too and that it can be equally distressing. Although I am extremely grateful that I gained so many friends in this yearlong journey, I am completely heartbroken over the friendships that I also lost.

In my pre-cancer existence, it was extremely rare that I wasn't the life of the party, the magnet, the Energizer Bunny, the comedian, the storyteller. With energy to spare, I had never experienced *not* being that person. With cancer however, I learned all about "fair weather friends." To my dismay, a few friends that I really cared for, who I thought in return really cared for me, just didn't show up. They showed their true colours when I was no longer healthy. I decided not only did I severely dislike a one-sided friendship, but I also chose not to invest in it anymore.

Some days, when I had too much time on my hands while sick in bed, my thoughts returned to those "friends." It angers me a bit now, as I shouldn't have had to even worry about why they hadn't called or texted as I laid there, so incredibly ill. But I did worry about it, because it hurt and they really mattered to me, their absence such an inconceivable mystery. I had invested a great deal of myself in those friendships over the past several years and I mistakenly assumed that while I was basically dying and desperately needing support, they, in turn, would be there for me. I realized that when I stopped being able to give them the care and time *they* needed, they simply fell out of the picture, unable to maintain a relationship. What bothered me the most about their absence was that I truly thought I meant something to them, and their silence confirmed that I actually didn't.

One of these "fair weather friends" texted me one day and said, "I've known about your cancer for six months, but I haven't reached out because I didn't know what to say." *Imagine.* I politely thanked him for his honesty, explained that in future you simply say, "I know you are unwell and that you feel like crap. It totally sucks and I am here for you." Truly, not rocket science. And then, thinking about the fact that I no longer had time for people who either couldn't handle facing my illness or didn't have the skills to try to connect, I blocked him.

Knowing that true friends are there in good times *and* in bad allowed me to do some "housecleaning." It bothered me a great deal, but time is precious, and I don't have time now for people who can't reciprocate the efforts of a true friendship. And although I realize many people won't fully ever grasp how truly awful this whole battle was for me, as I hid it well, nevertheless, cancer is cancer, and no matter how much it "appears" that things are okay, *true* friends will *always* insist on checking in to make sure things really are okay.

My besties checked in on the regular. Sometimes weeks would go by before I could see them again, as I refused to see anyone when I was at my lowest, but they texted and called and asked how I was doing and how my appointments went, often.

Many times Shannon would show up with a coffee or a tea and a little treat for me, and I would do my best to get a bit of lipstick on or to get up out of bed and painfully get to the couch, still refusing to be seen at my most vulnerable. On the days when I couldn't get out of bed, she would visit me in my bedroom, and she'd sit crammed up in a little space in an uncomfortable chair and watch over me. Occasionally we sat down by the beach if I was well enough to make it back up the hill. On one of those visits, I really struggled. I still remember that day so clearly. My chemo-affected heart was beating wildly in my chest. I was gasping for breath and felt quite dizzy with each step. I could only walk one step at a time and then I would lean heavily over my walking stick, seeing stars and almost fainting as my body worked hard to adjust to the change in elevation. I slowly made the climb back up the hill to our house, with Shannon protectively standing behind me in case I collapsed or lost my balance and fell. I had atrophied leg muscles that wobbled and shook as I hoisted myself along. That particular day, there was no hiding just how unwell I was, but I celebrated that at least I was outside, and grateful for my dear friend.

Tracy would come visit and a few times offered to massage my aching shoulders. It was awkward with my wig and hat, so even though I felt completely vulnerable, I removed them. She reassured me that she didn't mind touching my bald head. Her massage and her acceptance both gave me great relief even though I felt embarrassed and worried that my bald head was totally unpleasant. I could feel her hands shaking with emotion as she massaged me, taking my aches away and proving that I was still touchable.

Knowing these dear friends were this loving was so very comforting to me. A lifetime of friendship raising our kids together made it so I was comfortable enough with Shannon and Tracy that they could see me feeling quite poorly, but no one but Mike ever saw me at my absolute worst.

When I was too sick to visit, my amazing friends made the long drive out and left soup at my door and didn't see me at all. These many generous acts of kindness were definitely the mark of true friendship.

It was also hard to feel like I had missed out on so much over the past year. Dinner parties, golfing, guitar lessons and jams, hosting events, travel, sailing, kayaking, skiing—all of the social things I truly loved—fell by the wayside. I fell behind in all aspects of my friends' lives—birthdays, trips, anniversaries, graduations, family celebrations—and I was greatly aware that life indeed continued on without me. I was sad when I knew my friends were doing things without me, sadder still when I didn't know at all.

Oftentimes people would make decisions for me, to protect me. They would choose only to visit for an hour, so I wouldn't get tired out and they decided not to visit too often, in fear of bringing germs in the house. I was however, lonely, fighting boredom, and in need of support. Sometimes I struggled with what to say about it all and I discovered the delicate dance of communication and self-assertion.

I also found I became leery of people asking, "How are you doing?" I didn't know how to answer. What did they really want to hear? If I skipped over things, I sounded dismissive, but if I really tried to talk, I watched their eyes glaze over.

I decided to connect with another update, as the texts and emails were still regularly coming in.

Social Media Post #18
September 21

♡ Hi my dear friends ♡

So nice to have so many check-ins. People have asked me lately how I'm feeling, what's next in recovery, and when will I know if my cancer is gone. I'm feeling like I've been through the wring cycle of an old washing machine . . . beat up and tired; but sooooo happy to be finished treatments. Each day I try to walk outside a little bit but it's definitely at a snail's pace. By lunch I'm ready for a nap, lol. Some days I think I have little fuzzies of hair sprouting back, but I'm basically still bald. ☺ It's so weird!

The cancer was removed with the full hysterectomy, and the chemo and radiation was to fry off any rogue cells, but ultimately I've been told the only way to know that all of the treatments have worked is if it never comes back. So that is sort of a mind-bender, but if I don't get cancer within the next five years then they will officially say I'm back to status quo with all other women my same age.

I continue to have unexplained fevers that we are trying to sort through, but my golly if I can stay away from emerg I certainly will.

Slowly thinking about playing the guitar again, and just yesterday managed to go by myself to Sobeys for a few grocery items. That was a huge deal!

Anyhow, that is all for now. I continue to marvel at just how amazing and supportive you all are, and I am grateful for each and every one of you.

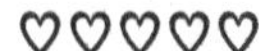

39

ANNIE AND MADDIE AND THE RINGING OF THE BELLS

My dear daughters were slowly starting to adjust to the fact that the worst was now over. They too had been holding their breath and worried for close to a year. I tried my best to always have a hat or a wig on when they were coming to visit as I truly couldn't bear the thought of them seeing me looking so awful; I certainly refused to let them see me any worse, when I already felt so weak and so vulnerable. No child, even as an adult, needs to see their mother bald, moaning, and in bed. It's just too much.

Sometimes, they would unexpectedly connect on a video call, and I would scramble to get a hat on my head before I answered, but at times I would be too sick to make the effort to cover my baldness, and those times I really, truly hated. They smiled through it all and told me it was fine, but I still don't know if they were being polite or honestly didn't mind—perhaps a bit of both.

Even sick in bed, I did my best to still be their mama. I'd ask how they were doing and I'd try to keep up with the ins and outs of young adulthood—friendships, parties, careers, house issues, meal prep, cleaning, groceries, roommates, boyfriends, and university, to name a few. I missed them both so much. I missed being able to hug and squeeze them in great big mama-bear hugs. I went several weeks at a time not seeing them. They feared, as did I, that they might bring a bug in the house, being active young people.

As the days wore on, they continued to check in and to manage their lives beautifully while I was struggling with mine; in some ways it was bittersweet, as I realized they were actually grown-ups and didn't need to be mothered. As every mother does, I longed for the days that we were all under one roof; I missed those days terribly, yet at the same time and in such stark contrast, I was very grateful they were grown up and could at least process my illness a little better than if they were younger. In some ways I was glad they didn't see me every day, so I could hide how truly sick I was. I still had a long road ahead.

Time continued to slowly pass and as the air changed, fall approached. Acquiring days with no need for more treatment or hospitals, felt wonderful. One day in September, roughly two weeks after I had been discharged, Mike invited me to go over to the family cottage for an hour to visit his dad. I agreed to go as I wanted both a change of scenery and to attempt a small walk on the flat, grassy property.

We had a little visit there, and I walked about two hundred yards. I was so happy! It was a tremendous accomplishment. Flashbacks of staggering five feet from bedroom to bathroom crossed my brain. Struggling to even just get into the car or walk my driveway seemed all too recent, yet here I was, able to slowly, carefully make a wee bit of progress. Breathless, sweaty, and quickly tuckered out, I told Mike I was good to go back to our home. Mike looked distracted for some reason, and stalled us. I couldn't understand why, and my patience was challenged as I needed to get back to resting. We said goodbye to Mike's dad and headed back to our place. As we pulled into the driveway, I heard bells ringing. Many. And cheers. *What on earth?*

And then I saw it. All of my dear friends, standing outside of our home, ringing bells, holding balloons, cheering, clapping, and smiling. My heart exploded. I burst into happy tears. I was amazed and in awe of this great gathering. I got out of the car and just stood there, speechless. They all continued smiling and ringing those bells, still clapping and cheering. "Congrats,

Andrea!" they called out. "You're done! Woo hoo!" I looked back at Mike. He stood there, beaming. This was quite a surprise. They all knew that with the earlier end of chemo, my original hope for ringing the big brass bell at the cancer centre hadn't materialized, and Mike and Shannon arranged this great moment of celebration. Tears poured down my face as I said, "I never rang the bell. I never rang the bell!"

Tracy came over and put a tiny bell in my hands and said, "Let's put an end to that right now! Ring the bell!" and I held on to that little clinky bell for dear life and shook it hard. Of course it wasn't the big brass bell that I'd planned on ringing, but it was still a wonderful moment; and maybe, it was even better this way.

The music teacher in me took over and I quickly organized my friends into a line and conducted them. As I pointed at each person to ring their bell, the melody revealed itself and people started humming along. I chuckled as I finished conducting "For She's a Jolly Good Fellow!" They all laughed at me, probably wondering if I was officially crazy.

The Nova Scotia weather was perfect that early September afternoon and we sat out, ocean-side, eating fruit salad and crackers with cheese as a few people drank beer. I felt a little self-conscious with the many eyes on me as I answered various questions and tried to keep up with the rapid conversations. It was a lot to focus on after so many months of ill health and solitude.

As I sat there with our friends, a feeling of freedom started to form in my soul. I looked at my sweet husband and thought about our upcoming trip; we were starting to accept the reality that we were finally through the treatment nightmare. The surprise celebration was a lovely sign-off to all that our tumultuous journey had entailed, and I finally felt like it was time to focus on healing and recovery. Friends and family continued to chat for a while longer about various things, and I was beyond grateful to discover that Marianne and Sue had very kindly weeded my Healing Garden. I was not well enough to tend to it just yet, and the weeds had accumulated quickly with the sunshine and perfect conditions for growth on the property.

A short while later, the gathering departed. I was sad to see people leave but knew it was the right thing for them to do as I was still very weak and needed rest. Feeling drained but with an immensely happy heart, I slept well that night.

A few weeks later, our thoughts shifted to Thanksgiving as it was my annual tradition to host a full turkey dinner for a crowd. (I'd been doing so for the past twenty-five years and with Mike together for the past seventeen.) Although I honestly never imagined we'd be able to host again, we decided we were going to uphold the tradition once more; come hell or high water. I was only six weeks post hospital discharge and still working through a great deal. Lara, once again, flew home and surprised me. She was a huge help and made cranberry sauce, a sweet potato casserole and two beautiful pumpkin pies.

As people arrived I kept returning to the outdoors to catch my breath and steady myself. It was an exquisite fall day. I revelled in the smell of the crisp, colourful leaves and was delighted to have a house full of happy people once again. I silently listed what I was most grateful for; my recovery (which was still a huge work in progress) for my family and friends so very present on the journey, and eternally grateful for each new day I get to have.

While outside, Mike's Aunt Jo and her husband, Hans, arrived. She quickly came up to me, her blue eyes wide and a grin even wider, "Andrea! The positive energy of this place! I could feel it as I drove up the driveway. There is some good juju happening here." I was deeply struck by this and recalled all over again that fateful day just a year prior that I had discovered the property and felt the same magical energy. I looked at her happily and whispered, "Kismet!"

"Look! Look! Look!" Mom suddenly hollered from the other room. I made my way as quickly as I could. "There's a huge eagle flying right outside your window! He's been hovering in the air, peering in."

My heart soared as I looked up and saw this great, regal, gigantic and powerful bird floating, suspended by air currents. He and I made eye contact, and it was as if he'd been looking for me. *You did it,* I heard him say. And he flew off with one quick, graceful movement. *Kismet, indeed.*

40

LYMPHEDEMA OR . . . NO?

The thing about lymphedema is, I might have it. I'm not sure if I *actually* do, or even when it started, but I have been in a lot of pain, and throughout my journey I have had medical people tell me I look really bloated. Puffy face, swollen fingers and abdomen, very sore legs with puffy skin on my calves. So one night in my many hours of googling about the still painful lump in my abdomen and my symptomatic congestion, I came across lymphedema. Basically it's when your lymphatic system is not functioning at its best and you get puffy and fluid-y. Doing my due diligence, I looked up a lymphatic massage specialist and found one with decent reviews. He was insistent that I needed to order and wear a full-body support hose, immediately. This hose would go from my toes all the way up to my bra line. "But," I pleaded in alarm, "I'm going to Florida in three weeks!"

"There's time," he said. "We will order it today."

"No, you don't understand, I'm going for peace of mind and recovery. You want me to wear a full-body support hose in the heat and on the beach??"

"Hmm." He thought for a moment and smiled. "Wear it at night, in your hotel room."

Say whaaaat? With a big fat "Nope," I promptly hopped off the table and quickly left.

The following week I saw another pelvic floor specialist for my various pelvic issues. I had capri pants on in our first meeting, and within the first five minutes, she said, "I see you have some lymphedema going on in your legs."

I was surprised. "How can you tell?"

"Well, not only am I a trained osteopath, acupuncturist, and pelvic floor therapist, I am also a lymphatic massage specialist."

I couldn't believe it. I explained about the first guy I'd seen, and she was very bothered by my story. She said, "You can't wear support hose. Your skin is still too sensitive from chemo and radiation and we don't even know if your heart can handle that much compression." I felt relieved and validated that I had just dodged a major bullet. She worked on me and massaged the lymph nodes on my back, my chest, my legs and deftly moved some fluid.

Shortly after that visit, I had a specialist appointment with oncology. Again I was disappointed that it was not my regular oncologist, the amazing Dr. Scott. Along with the "new" doc was an intern doctor in attendance. When the intern asked me if I had any questions, I asked him what I should be doing about my lymphedema.

"What?" he said, in surprise. "You don't have lymphedema."

I explained that two lymphatic specialists said I had it. He looked at my legs and pushed down hard on my skin. I yelped in pain.

"Nope. No lymphedema."

"How can you be sure?" I asked.

He explained that if I had it, my leg would keep an imprint of his thumb where he had pushed. I in no way wanted to dispute this highly educated man, and I respected the years of study he had committed to, but I did read in my own searches that the skin does not pit in the *early* stages of lymphedema. I knew I was likely in the mild stage, and I was desperate to prevent it developing into something more serious, but was not about to argue.

Two days later I attended an appointment with my family doctor, and I mentioned that I was told by two lymphatic specialists that I should be flying with compression socks. She made an appointment with the office nurse to take measurements and check my blood pressure on both arms and both ankles. Twenty minutes later I was handed a piece of paper with a prescription for 40–50mmHg compression socks. I was told that based on the numbers, I clearly had lymphedema and it was also determined that I needed to go back on my blood pressure meds. I was now in a bit of a state as our Florida trip was just three days away. Before I even drove home, I began calling everywhere only to discover that no one carried that gauge of sock.

"Is this an unusual sock?" I asked at the fifth place I called.

"Why yes. We *never* order that heavy a gauge."

I hung up and full panic set in as I mentally counted the hours left in the business day to find the right socks before my flight. My mind returned to my oddly and very swollen legs the year before, coming home from the Chris Stapleton concert that never was. Off I went to the drugstore. I figured I would buy compression socks over the counter so I'd at least have something; I mean, something is better than nothing, right? At the drug store, I headed to the home health care area. The woman I spoke with said, "Oh! Did you just call here a while ago?"

I actually couldn't remember if I had, as in total I had called fourteen stores. "Likely, yes," I replied, feeling a little sheepish.

She went out back to get another lady. That lady looked me slowly up and down looking quite perturbed. "Who did your measurements? Why do you need the socks? Can I examine your legs?" She explained that she'd been working there for over twenty years doing fittings and never once before had she had to order that heavy a compression sock. She looked really worried and felt that I should not be ordering them. She told me to call my doctor again and to double-check the information. I did. The information was correct. So she got out a checklist and asked me to review it. It said I would be a candidate for this gauge if I had severe fluid buildup, raw, ulcerated skin, etc.

"Hmph," I said, "that isn't me."

So we agreed to order the next gauge down. She thought they should arrive in time for the flight but that they perhaps might not, so I also bought an even lower 20–30 gauge over the counter just to be safe. I was told to wear the socks a few hours each morning to get used to them.

And so, I struggled fervently with those darn socks and ultimately needed Mike to power through and hoist them up to my knee. I watched in awe and tried not to giggle as he grunted and groaned and pushed and wiggled. *Good Lord, how do seniors manage these things all on their own?* I wore them dutifully for a few hours and then had to get Mike to take them off. This was Saturday. I wore them on Sunday too. On Monday I got a call that my special order was in, and Mike went to pick them up. He brought them back and I tried to get them on. Keep in mind, this is now the 30–40 gauge, not even the originally recommended 40–50 gauge, and for the love of God, I was on my back, on my front, upside down, and had my feet almost over my head as Mike tried to get those darn things on. I watched in fascination as he turned pink, then red, then purple, gasping and sputtering and sweating as he worked at getting the socks on. After five minutes of this, we had managed to only get one sock halfway over my foot. Shortly thereafter, we quit. In summary:

- One lymphatic specialist said I needed full-body hose.
- One lymphatic specialist said absolutely no hose, but yes to knee socks.
- Oncology doc said no need for anything, I don't have lymphedema.
- Nurse at the family doctor's office said yes, based on the measurements and readings by her machine, I do indeed have lymphedema and that I was to get the heaviest gauge of socks, special order.
- Home health care lady said no way, do NOT get the heaviest gauge.

You can see how confusing and upsetting all of this was with so many conflicting assessments. Once again, the health care system had really let me down.

41
FLORIDA

This time, packing for Florida looked a little different. I smiled in amusement at the prioritized items; we were indeed aging. First to go in my bag was the digital thermometer, the blood pressure machine, extra compression socks, my big, boofy beach hat for my still very bald head, a gigantic one-piece bathing suit, and of course, the dilator. A bag of meds included blood pressure pills, bladder pills, Restoralax, Tylenol, Ativan, Benadryl, magnesium, fish oil, and eye drops. Then of course my orthotic sandals, a 60 SPF sunblock, all of my electronics—my carry-on was filled to overflowing before I even had a single "regular" clothes item packed. I can tell you, this year, a bikini was nowhere in sight. A familiar Bob Dylan song popped into my head as I stared at the mountain of stuff in the suitcase. *For the tiiimes . . . they are a-chaaaangin'.*

We made it to beautiful Naples after a long day of travel, and I was overjoyed and greatly relieved that we had arrived without any major delays or issues. However, even with the requested wheelchair that was booked for travel throughout the three airports, I found I was still deeply exhausted; it was more walking, lugging, and energy than I had expended in well over a year. We got to the condo at nine thirty that night, and I happily had Mike peel off my 20–30-gauge compression socks. I was pleased to see that this time, I had no swelling. I crashed face first on the sofa only minutes after arrival and fell quickly to sleep.

The next day we got a load of groceries and relaxed by the pool for several hours. It was exactly what we needed. My mind nervously wandered, though, as I thought about my nether regions. Again, a lonely path of confusion and worry, to walk alone. I constantly sought answers and needed more information than I could easily find. I still had extensive damage in all pelvic areas and needed reassurance from other radiation folk that I would eventually heal. I decided to reach out as an anonymous member in my online Chemo Support group.

Social Media Post:
November 1

> Ladies, let's talk about sex . . . I've read that pelvic radiation can
> ultimately lead to fractured pelvic bones. I've gone through a
> hysterectomy, chemo, and radiation. I have vaginal stenosis
> happening. I'm terrified to have sex, but with the surgery and the
> treatments, it's been a year, and I feel like it's time to "get back on
> the horse," so to speak. My poor husband. I'm thinking, how do I
> explain the delicacies of sex to him after all I have been through
> and how my body has changed? "Okay, hunny. Don't pound
> me too vigorously or you'll crack my pelvis, and not too deeply
> or it'll really hurt . . . Don't touch my stomach as my scar tissue
> and nerve damage is really sensitive, oh and try not to squish
> my legs or rest yours on them in any position because of my
> lymphedema. And, lastly but most importantly, be careful of my
> external hemorrhoids . . ." Is there ANYONE who can relate? Is
> sex even possible?

Anxiously I waited and it was only moments before the comments piled in. The confidential feedback that I received was both terrifying and hilarious. I now know at least I am not alone in this worrisome problem, but even still, no better off.

During that first week, we worked our way through some of my "Things to see and do" list, one of which was to visit The Cheesecake Factory. As we crossed the parking lot in the Florida heat, I was greatly aware of my painful, swollen body. Even though the compression socks had prevented additional swelling while flying, I still had much pain and moderate swelling throughout my entire frame. Crossing the large parking lot was a challenge in and of itself, and my speed could best be described as "slower than a senior sloth's pace."

I truly believe that in that moment of more struggle and humility, the universe intervened and dropped an opportunity in for some humour.

I could hear music blaring from the outdoor speakers near the entrance to The Cheesecake Factory. As the song became more audible, I realized it was one of my favorite tunes, Girl from Ipanema. I slowly bobbed my bald head under my big white beach hat, listening to the familiar, happy tune. As I struggled along with my painful, swollen legs and feet, my mind raced and I started laughing while new lyrics came to me.

Short and fat and old and jiggly, the girl with lymphedema goes walking, and when she passes, each one she passes goes aww! I began to laugh harder. *Yes! Those would make great play on words. I'll call the song, "Girl with Lymphedema."* As I continued to slowly make my way, I could hear in my head more new lyrics to the song. *Bald like that, she's sore but wiggly, the flu-id in her knees so jiggly, and when she passes, each one she passes goes aww!* I could not stop laughing at how enjoyable these new words were, and I'm willing to bet my music-loving friends will appreciate the parody. "Girl from Ipanema" is a famous jazz song; a fantastic tune. Put it this way—if you don't know it after you look it up, we can't be friends anymore.

The Florida days slowly passed as Mike and I continued to lap up sunshine and laze by the pool. We were so very grateful to finally have no more stress and no more treatments. The one-year anniversary of my cancer diagnosis was fast approaching, and I started to think about how I wanted to mark the day. I wanted to do something fun, distracting, so I wouldn't replay in my mind the nightmare of a year ago, quite honestly one of the worst days of my life. I explored a few options—a nurturing spa event, an entertaining water park, a trip to the zoo, perhaps—but as the time neared, none of the ideas felt right, and truthfully, I didn't have the energy anyway.

And then it came to me; I would go to the beach and be restored by the ocean. The ocean is one of my all-time favourite places on the planet, and I recognized that I could symbolically and physically wash away my torment and be free to cry, scream, laugh, and be present for whatever emotions came up. I planned to jump into the water precisely at eleven a.m., the exact time the hammer had dropped on me the year before. Mike accompanied me to the beach, and it was an emotional time for us both. I knew I'd made the right choice as I swam and dove and cried tears of heartache and also of joy. I was grateful to be in the warm sun, and the fresh, gentle breeze washed much of the heavy emotions away. We ended the day with a beautiful steak dinner, and I started envisioning my future with a healthier lifestyle and more energy.

The next two weeks went by in a blur of naps, writing, very slow walks to the beach, sunsets, much time poolside, fine food, a few brief shopping excursions, TV watching, and barbeques. It was a relaxing, stress-free, beautiful time for us together.

Sadly, the stenosis greatly affected my plans for any intimacy, and I questioned whether I needed a different apparatus; I didn't feel I was making much progress with the current tool.

"Is there a sex shop in Naples?" I asked one morning over breakfast.

Mike nearly spat out his mouthful of coffee. "I doubt it," he said. "This is a pretty upscale place."

Immediately he began searching on his phone and located a place called Jack and Jill's Couples Shop. We drove over and sat there awkwardly in the car watching various odd types come and go with discreet, black plastic purchase bags. We had a good laugh knowing we were the next weirdos about to go in, a middle-aged couple looking for a dildo, one of us bald and wearing a giant beach hat.

We got ready, then Mike decided to play a little joke on me. He announced he was staying in the car. I certainly did *not* want to go in by myself. I glanced in the back seat and saw my bright red wig, which I had tossed behind in the heat a few days earlier. I handed it to Mike, trying to smooth over any more anxious feelings. "Here, wear this," I teased, and he put it on and proceeded to get out of the car. It looked hilarious with his big bushy beard and manly face, and he started to walk over to the entrance. I painfully doubled over laughing hysterically in the parking lot. He had relieved our awkward situation and had me in stitches once again. (For the record, he did not go into the shop wearing my wig, although I secretly wished he had.)

We spent a great deal of time in the store, shocked and fascinated by all that we saw there. We ultimately made a purchase that seemed more human-like than the pink, narrow-tipped dilator, in hopes I could make more progress in the "sealed vault" department. Sadly, things still did not return to normal. I learned that with this level of severe damage it can take up to a full year of regular work and that the scary fact is, some people *never* fully recover.

Even with the awfully disappointing continued pelvic issues, we still managed to have a great vacation. The sunshine and good vibes healed us in many ways and the three weeks flew by. We wrapped up a lovely time and headed to the airport, feeling rested and ready to begin a new chapter back home in Nova Scotia.

As our bags went through the scanners at the airport, I left Mike and moved to a bench off to the side to put my boots back on. It took a bit of time and effort as they were new and stiff. As I struggled, I anxiously looked over my shoulder to check on the progress of the security line. Across the crowd, I saw Mike's face and could tell something was up. He looked around, eyes searching, until he found me. He mouthed, "Andrea, come here," his hands beckoning. I took in the scene before me. Mike looked expectant, slightly amused, and mildly concerned; a male TSA agent was standing still, waiting with him, also looking at me with an odd look on his face. I saw that my bag had been selected to be searched. I hobbled over as best I could, my boots still only half on my feet.

The agent looked at me; he was holding my new carry-on. Loudly and firmly he inquired, "Ma'am, is this your bag?"

"Yes!" I replied, pleasantly and excitedly, thinking of all the Christmas presents I'd purchased, now in said carry-on. I had carefully wrapped them all in packing paper, as they were delicate and breakable.

"So you are aware of the contents of this bag, and its contents are all yours?" he continued.

I wasn't sure why I would possibly be getting a bag search, so I tried not to look nervous. Thinking of the gifts and not wanting to risk anything being held up or damaged, I made even bigger efforts to look cheery and confident. I imagined Christmas morning, handing out the gifts—cinnamon-scented soaps, nutcrackers, new clothes—and I innocently replied once more, smiling brightly with even more exuberance, while trying to explain the gifts. "Yes, this is my bag and it is filled with super fun things."

As far as the agent was concerned, I had responded with too much excitement. I couldn't understand now why he looked at me like I was either crazy or a total horny pervert. I looked straight at him, trying to interpret his expressions.

"So, it's okay if I search the bag then?" He looked awkward, apologetic, but sort of like he was trying not to smile.

Mike stood there making great efforts not to laugh. I looked from one face to the other, not understanding the expressions. Behind me, lines of people were waiting to get through and now looking down the line to see why there was a hold-up. It hadn't yet occurred to me what was going on. I was looking the agent square in the eye and hadn't yet looked at the screen.

I watched as he snapped on the blue plastic gloves and went through my carry-on, carefully unzipping the middle layer, picking up the wrapped items and examining all of them. And then I saw it. The brightly coloured member, front and centre. I had forgotten that my new medical apparatus—okay, the dildo, a.k.a. The "Floridian Special"—was in there.

The night before I had packed three different bags—a suitcase to be checked, the carry-on, and my large purse. I had moved several things around to get everything to fit. And then it dawned on me that not only was it there for the agent to see, this private item was now up on the *giant X-ray screen*. Clear as day, my dildo would be visible for *all* to see.

The TSA guy looked up at Mike and likely thought, *Great, does her husband know she travels with a dildo?* or worse, did he think, *this couple is pretty into their toys!* Mike stood there, taking it all in, secretly wishing he could take a picture of the now enlarged item on full display.

With adrenalin building I looked up at the giant X-ray and could see several muddled grey items. My eyes continued to briefly search and then right smack in the middle of the screen, clearly visible, life-like head and all, the item causing the awkward exchange—the seven-and-a-half-inch beast! Bigger still on the giant screen. *Oh gosh.* I breathed deeply and slowly turned to look at the lineup of people behind me. I saw them all smiling, looking directly at me. I turned to Mike, my blushing face a combination of embarrassment and horror, just as he started to full-out laugh at me. He leaned into my ear and whispered, "You're a piece of work."

The agent finally turned around, facing me as I avoided eye contact. I sheepishly accepted my bag as he handed it back to me, saying, "Have a nice day, ma'am."

42

IS THIS IN OUR VOWS?

It's not very often that a wife sees her husband walking around with a seven-and-a-half-inch, lubed up dildo, but one night that's exactly what I saw. Let me clarify. I am still dealing with pelvic issues and have been instructed by oncology that I must use the vaginal dilator three times a week for at least a year. *Oh joy*, you think? Sadly, no, it is definitely not "joy"; it is a very painful process, wretchedly necessary and horribly worrisome when one knows that the effects of radiation can last up to (and sometimes more than) twelve months' post-radiation.

On this particular December night, I was watching TV and my alarm went off, reminding me to go do my due diligence. I quietly excused myself and went to the bedroom in the lower part of the house, only to discover two problems. One, it was exceptionally cold down there, and two, Duey was completely stretched out, asleep, hogging the entire king-sized bed. I didn't want to deal with being frozen during the unpleasantries, nor did I want to do this next to our furry, drooly, two-hundred-pound beast.

I decided to go back up to the main floor to use a different location. Off I went, wriggling out of my pants and laying out a protective towel over the sheets. I lubed up the dildo. This is quite necessary, as the vaginal walls are so damaged from radiation that one wouldn't make much progress otherwise. I turned the dial to get the vibrations started, and again, you would think this would be not too bad a task, but the vibrations are in an attempt to break down scar tissue. It's actually awful and I have to do it every second day. So I turn it on and to my surprise, nothing happens; it doesn't hum in the slightest. *Ugh. The batteries must be dead.* So, up I get (which in itself these days is a lot of work) and with lubed-up dildo in hand (I can't lay it down or it'll get lint fuzzies and dog hairs on it), I quietly sneak out of the bedroom wearing only my top, to wander around, looking for batteries.

I find some rechargeable ones and return to the room. I carefully balance the dildo between my pinky and ring finger so I can use both hands to gently twist off the cover to replace the batteries, only to discover they are the wrong size. I exhale deeply. *Are you kidding me?* So, I awkwardly manoeuvre out of bed yet again and go search for some more batteries, hoping to find the right size. I find them, insert them, and … nothing. It's completely dead. I can feel myself losing patience. "Are these batteries charged?" I call from the bedroom, clearly hearing my own annoyance.

I get out of bed a third time and go back to the living room, the dildo discreetly behind my back.

"Yes," Mike says, looking at me and wondering why I am asking about batteries.

I go back to the bedroom, quickly losing what little enthusiasm I barely had. I look to see which end of the battery to insert first and then realize I can't see the little "+" and "-" signs without my glasses. *Lord, give me patience.* I sigh this time with an even deeper exhale, trying to avoid overreacting as my body stiffens and my shoulders rise. I struggle out of bed again (now the *fourth* time) to retrieve my glasses, only to find that in typical dog fashion, Duey has awoken from his slumber downstairs and has now decided to take over *this* bed.

Firmly I tell him to "Get off the bed." In reply he snores deeply and loudly. Now, getting a sleeping Duey off the bed is no easy task, and I have to use both hands to pull on his front legs. With the need to use *both* hands, I look around, trying to figure out where to put the lubed-up dildo. On the bed? No, even more dog hairs. I step over my carefully folded clothes pile and move to place the tool carefully on the dresser and realize that, ironically, it won't "stand up" on its own as the floors are slightly uneven. I could rest it on the windowsill and lean it against the glass, but the window ledge is about one centimetre too narrow for the base. I think for a minute, and in desperation to get the job done, I carefully place it . . . *ugh* . . . in my MOUTH. I bite down on the thing to keep it in place as it teeters and bounces around freely like a very happy dog wagging its very large tail. "C'mon Duey." I say, in a garbled sort of way, my jaw now stretched wide open as the fondly nicknamed "Floridian Special" happens to have a good diameter. Still biting it between my teeth and trying not to drop it, in a garbled sort of way I shout, "GET . . . OFF . . . THE . . . BED!"

I drag Duey to the floor and he grumbles a bit. I lie down now huffing and puffing and put my glasses on to see how to put the batteries in. For some weird reason, the batteries don't fit even though they are the correct size. I give a little push and get one in. Then I insert the other one only to discover it's the wrong way around. It gets stuck. *What the actual hell! Why is this so bloody difficult?* I have lost count of the number of times I've had to climb out of bed. The clean towel is now on the floor, the bed sheets are twisted up like a cinnamon bun, and Duey is panting and drooling on my discarded clothing.

I go back to the living room, still in just my shirt and no bottoms, still holding the lubed-up dildo, and walk over to my husband. His eyebrows rise and a smile crosses his face as he takes me in. I yell, "I got the batteries jammed in my stupid dildo and I can't get them out!" I am beyond annoyed by this point. I pass it to him. "Be careful of the lube," I add as an afterthought.

He can't place his hands around the thing because of the all the lube and therefore can't get any leverage to pull out the batteries. He groans, as now he has to get up and go downstairs to the basement to get needle-nosed pliers and maybe the vice grips.

I stand there rocking back and forth mumbling, "This is my life . . . this is my *actual* life" in a mantra, trying to calm down.

Mike comes back upstairs and hands me the dildo. "Try this," he says half smiling and adds, "Our lives are crazy." *Oh mister, you don't even know the half of it.*

I go back to the bedroom trying to muster up any enthusiasm at all for this mundane task, and unbelievably, the darn thing STILL won't turn on. I am now officially losing my mind. I get up *again* and go out to the living room and hand it to him. "It still won't turn on!" I yell even louder now.

Mike looks totally perturbed and then suddenly it dawns on him that the rechargeable batteries don't have quite enough power to run the vibrator. He gets up and goes upstairs this time.

After a few minutes, trying hard to wait patiently but not getting any update, I call up to him. "What are you doing now?" I start to feel guilty for the annoyance and volume of my voice.

"Looking for regular batteries," he replies, also sounding more than a little vexed. A few minutes go by. "Can I take them out of your Christmas village?" he calls down.

Oh. My. Dear. God. My life. Big breath, Andrea. Biiiig breath. "If you must," I answer, thinking over and over that we really should have our own TV show by now.

He comes back with the batteries and takes the dildo from me carefully, delicately squeezing the tip with thumb and finger this time, still trying not to get lube all over his hands. He disappears to the basement again to take the rechargeable batteries out and put the regular ones in. He comes back up the stairs carefully holding the impressive, lubed-up member by its tip and walks toward me, grinning. It was quite a sight, and I burst in to complete fits and giggles. He handed me the dildo, and *finally* I got the job done.

After I'd finished and replayed the ridiculous events in my mind, I pictured an announcer with a microphone, handing an award to Mike, saying, *Congratulations to Mike Ritcey, a well-seasoned individual in these mighty fine moments of life.* And then I recalled a somewhat similar event from several years past.

Mike's parents visited their condo in Florida several times a year and would often leave clothing and other frequently used items there as they regularly travelled back and forth. On one occasion, Mike and I were vacationing with them, and they flew home a few days before us. Mike received a phone call from his mother shortly after she'd unpacked. She had forgotten something.

He hung up the phone from their quick conversation and started laughing, looking a little awkward. "Great. Just great," he said to me.

"What is it?" I asked, a little worried.

"I have to bring my mom's boob back." She had had breast cancer in her mid-thirties and had a prosthetic breast made that she wore frequently. "Can you see it now? The alarms go off in customs and they search my carry-on and pull out the prosthetic, fleshy cone saying, 'What's this, sir?' and I say, 'Uh, that's my mom's boob.'"

I mentioned this memory to him after all of the dildo events. Between his mom's boob and my dildo, we've had some pretty funny experiences. *God love ya, my dear man. You are indeed my hero.*

43

AND A PARTRIDGE IN A PEAR TREE

It hit me one day. I was finished. Completely done with all the hell—the emotional turmoil and the physical trauma. No more treatments, no more hospitals, no more trips to emerg and no more frightening, unexpected, horrendously painful moments. Recovering from the PTSD could now be my focus, and I could begin to just . . . heal.

I started mentally checking off all that I was now finished. *So long, all you nurses who could not get a needle in me. Goodbye, amazing rad techs, receptionists, and doctors. See ya, thank-you notes, casseroles, and soups. Good riddance, bone pain, seven-pound clay babies, bladder accidents, diapers, disgusting liquid concoctions, phone calls, johnnie shirts, modified diets, broths, and shedding hair.* In awe, I thought about all that Mike and I had endured this past year and it played out like a familiar Christmas tune, "On the first day of treatment, my cancer brought to me, a very painful hysterectomy." *Ha.* I continued to think about all we'd been through. *If only there were twelve items to sing about in total like the song, instead of all of which came flying back. I tried to calculate numerically what our year was like.*

- 2,987,469,362 shed tears
- 13,096 boxes of Kleenex
- 325,873 blood tests

- 278,005 litres of consumed water
- 242, 554 steroids
- 516 sleepless nights
- 245 anti-nausea pills
- 25 pelvic radiations
- 16 pounds of Restoralax (more or less)
- 12 prescriptions for Ativan
- 11 trillion CT scans
- 10 boxes of Preparation H
- 9 prescriptions for hydromorphone
- 8 trips to emerg
- 7 million miles on the car
- 6 anti-coagulant punch needles
- 5 … rounds of chemo …
- 4 billion failed IV attempts
- 3 hospital admissions
- 2 brachytherapies
- And (sing it with me), "a partridge in a pear tree!"

44

LADIES AND GENTLEMEN, THE ONE . . . THE ONLY . . . MIKE RITCEY!!

And so, here we are. I made it. *We* made it. Looking back, I try to put my thoughts of it all into a succinct summary. I feel like somehow I was handed this horrible, unexpected chapter in the book of life, and yet I endured and rose to the top. I am stronger now. I have self-love and know my worth. I have a much tighter circle of friends, and my sister and I are a great deal closer. Mentally I have torn out and thrown away the pages from this past years' chapter. My exhaustive, horrendous year is now done. As I look back on this incredible journey, I am eternally grateful for the unwavering support of my dear husband. I truly feel he saved my life. Along with Dr. Scott, of course.

I was given an incredible gift the day I met Mike, so many years ago. I had been separated from the girls' dad for a year and wasn't sure how I felt about dating again. A mutual friend set us up, insisting we would be perfect for one another, and lo and behold, she was right.

Mike and I have been married for fourteen incredible years and together for eighteen. We have honestly laughed with each other every single day since that fateful first date. Our relationship started out as friends, and our love grew from there. I highly recommend marrying one's best friend. We have discovered that together, we can achieve anything we put our minds to; we can conquer all.

We've been through so very much as a couple—the cancer, of course, but not just mine; several other family in-law members have also dealt with this awful disease. We both have suffered the unspeakable loss of loved ones in tragically awful ways, and we managed to come through it. Our failed house dreams and the endless, exhausting, stressful, repeated cycle of purchasing, packing, moving, and selling over only just two years was incredibly frustrating and worrisome. Top it all off with several stressful jobs, raising a family, and much more. The strength of our marriage truly is a testament to our love and devotion to one another. They say if a couple can withstand a death, a move, a job loss, etc., they should be good. Well I'm pretty sure we can say, we're good!

I hope to never experience anything like this past year, ever again. As for my dear husband, no one should have to witness the pain and torment of an ill partner the way he did. I cannot imagine what it was like for him. He was there for me this year like no other, and through the horrors of it all, he was my rock. The countless, sometimes terrifying moments that he bravely, calmly, repeatedly dealt with for months on end were extremely difficult and oftentimes quite lonely.

He attended all the oncology appointments, most of the twenty-seven radiation sessions, and every trip to emerg. He accompanied me for all five chemo days, sitting for eight hours at a time in a horribly uncomfortable chair, and managed, through this entire ordeal, to continue working away at his job; he never once requested time off for stress leave. He played the role of nurse, dispensing my medicine and cleaning up vomit, assisting me in the shower, blow-drying my hair, and holding me up when I fainted. He brought me tea and meals and in general, continued watching over me Every. Single. Day.

And, amazingly, while working a full-time job with great responsibilities and caring for me, he single-handedly did all the housework—garbage and groceries, food prep and cooking, dishwashing and dog care, laundry, the care of all the indoor plants (of which we have many), the yard work through four seasons—plus all of the car appointments, and more.

It was a year of endless struggle and yet surprisingly, endless growth. Mike and I somehow managed to survive the year, and we are of course, still "thick as thieves." He remains my steadfast soldier, my beacon of hope in my darkest of hours. People marvel at how positive we remained through all of the hell; I credit my partner.

So, my darling. How could I not end this memoir without a tribute to you? As I think of our year together, I run a highlight reel in my mind:

- You putting my darn compressions socks on me. That in itself was a major workout.

- The ridiculous moment when you duct-taped my head (seems like forever ago). You were so tender and loving, trying to relieve my suffering. And also how you made that moment just so exceptionally humorous.

- The organizing of the ringing of the bells, knowing just what would cheer me. You are the most sentimental man.

- Driving me to the store in a race against time to get me some super-hold gel and hairspray for my mohawk.

- The memorable afternoon that I was feeling particularly unattractive—the five bright pink scars on my abdomen from the hysterectomy stretched out like number signs each the size of a quarter, my skin so pale on a surface that didn't look or feel like natural skin, my eyelashes and eyebrows all gone, and my head so hairless I resembled an egg. I said to you, "Do you ever just sit there and think what a freak show your wife is right now?" And without missing a beat you said, "Honey, I've thought that for fifteen years!" We both cracked up laughing, me at your obnoxious wit, and you because you enjoy our shocking banter and the reactions you get.

- The night I was really struggling in the horrendous weeks after my clay-baby ordeal, still too fresh from the hysterectomy to get into a twisted position to insert a suppository yet I couldn't stand the severe pain even a second longer. Desperate and embarrassed, I had to ask you for help. I lay there, feeling awful and exposed, and I started crying. I couldn't believe what my life had become. I turned to you and said, "I'm so sorry for all of this." and you cracked up laughing and said, "What are you talking about, this is fun!" And incredibly, in that horrible moment, you had me bursting out laughing, when I was at an all-time low, so utterly helpless and humiliated. You brought it home once again with humour and love, and I thank you for that.

- Pushing my heavy, rickety wheelchair through airports with all of our luggage and all that that entailed, bumping over awkward floors and ramps, struggling to get me through the long corridors to the plane. I had started to cry yet again, feeling frustrated and helpless and feeling badly for you as you struggled to carry the load, and you simply reached down and kissed my cheek to tell me it was all okay.

- The dildo we had to buy in Naples. Thank you for making the awkward trip to that shop so gosh-darn memorable.

- The endless nicknames—at my most-bald (baldilocks, egghead, cue ball, nipple head) and then as the hair came in (my little SOS pad, scrubby, scruffy, scratchy).

There are no words to describe my love and my gratitude for you, for us. Your commitment to me and your love for me knows no bounds. Your support and your stability on a daily basis kept me sane and truly allowed me to "fight the fight." You, too, lost a year of your life looking after me, and yet you gracefully carried the hardest role—the caregiver. Looking after someone you love and seeing them so ill is beyond stressful and is exceedingly challenging. You have been through so much, yet you just plug away and act like it was nothing. You are a man of incredible strength, love, devotion, and humour. I want the world to know how fabulous you are and how much I love you. When we took our vows, I never dreamed we'd have so many immense challenges. Our wedding vow "in sickness and in health" really was tested to its limits this year, and there is no one I would ever want to walk this path with but you.

I love you more than I ever knew I could. And now, we begin a new chapter, a new beginning, together, and I am ready.

EPILOGUE

"Time!" Mike yelled from the shoreline. Adrenalin pumping, I took the deepest breath I could muster and dove underwater with all my might. I opened my mouth and screamed a year's worth of anguish as loudly as my voice could possibly scream. My vocal chords burned with the force, but still, I continued. Finally, I felt free. I was swimming! I shook my head hard and spat out salty water. I pushed onward, diving deeper underwater, my legs kicking strong and fast as I pulled my arms through the powerful current as best I could. Feeling my lungs were about to burst, I allowed my body to slowly float back up to the surface, not quite ready to depart the underworld. My head emerged from the turquoise water and I felt the salt water leave my eyes while the burning sun shone brightly down on my bald head. I found my footing on the sandy ocean floor, and, fully above water now, mentally signed off on this year from hell.

Smiling, I began the journey back to the shore, rough pebbles scraping the soles of my feet. Today I begin to move forward, to heal in the warm southern sun, baptized by the ocean with dolphins and good vibes. I am, renewed.

THE END.

Andrea Leigh Ritcey

A "good ole, Nova Scotia girl," Andrea Leigh Ritcey was raised in a quaint little town just outside of Halifax, Nova Scotia. In 1994 she graduated from Acadia University with two degrees; Bachelor of Music and Bachelor of Education and went on to a near twenty-year career in the public school system. During this time, she worked with an accumulated total of close to 4000 students throughout the province conducting numerous bands, choirs and hosting many public performances. Outside of her career, she raised two amazing daughters, married the love of her life, opened up her own private music studio, held numerous recitals, sang in a regular choral group, recorded three CDs and went on to own a giant English Mastiff which she reared from puppyhood to 200-pound adult.

A musician, avid performer and community theatre actor, her favorite hobbies include golfing, down-hill skiing, gardening and interior decorating. Of the many shingles she could hang however, first and foremost would be "Teacher." It's in her heart, and in her soul. When her life went completely sideways with a cancer diagnosis, she realized, unquestionably, that she wanted to share her experiences in a memoir in order to help others. *I Never Rang the Bell* quickly materialized.

Currently Andrea resides in a small seaside village near "world famous" Peggy's Cove and is now in full recovery. She has returned to her students and continues to teach music to many. On any given day you can find her strumming her guitar or hanging out ocean-side with the loves of her life.

Acknowledgements

Inevitably, someone is going to read through this and feel like I missed them, and for that I am truly sorry. I have chemo brain; I'm only four months' post chemo after all. I am eternally grateful for every single act of kindness from every single one of you who connected with me. I love you all, with all of my heart. Thank you, eternally, for walking this path with me.

To Dr. Stephanie Scott: You, my dear, exemplify what a doctor truly needs to be to patients going through cancer. You are caring, reassuring, professional, kind, smart, on time, and so very patient. Your thoroughness and generous time spent answering all of our questions and allowing us to come to the best decisions together provided me with the ability to survive. I am alive because of you!

To Jeff Brown: You suggested I should write a book after I posted some ridiculous stories about this insane journey. Thank you for planting the seed and for giving me a voice.

To my social media friends: Your encouragement gave me a platform to tell my story with both humour and truth. Your support, cheers, and responses spurred me on toward a very positive mindset while I was so sick. Thank you for shaping me in this journey.

To my Alphas—Annie Comeau, Kimberly Dossett, Paula Minnikin, Emily Vincent, Sue Volcko: Your help and generous time was invaluable. Thank you so much for your very thoughtful feedback.

To my fellow warriors who walked their cancer journey in private: Thank you for reaching out to me. Advice about wigs, ideas for pain management and simply giving me hope was just what I needed. Thank you for walking alongside me.

To Alex Vodicka: You, my guiding light in the storm. How you had the strength to push through your own journey is beyond me. Thank you for always being there to answer my questions and to smooth my worries. You are a true friend. Sorry I keep forgetting to reply—chemo brain.

To my extended family—David (FIL), Simone, Janet (Shrubbie,) Gavin, Sara, Denis, Sue, Hans, and Jo: Your check-ins, your knowledge of this disease, your advice, and your confidence helped me more than you'll likely ever know. It was so helpful to know that I was not the first one in the family to walk this road. You already have either lived it or lived close to it, and your generous time given to me provided extra peace of mind.

To Marianne Ward: Thank you for completing my first edit. Your knowledge, patience and generosity are very much appreciated.

To Gwyneth Cristoffel: You are amazing and generous and super creative. Thank you for nailing the book cover. You make me feel extra proud!

To David Edelstein: Book formatting and also, my "manager" haha. Thank you for filling in the gaps with my many, many questions. You are patient and kind.

To Marina, Emily R., Jess and all of the staff at the Nova Scotia Cancer Centre: You continue on the daily to show up at your best and give your best each day to all. It makes a huge difference to the patients. (No one wants to go through this nightmare with a cranky staff.) You are special and you are amazing at your jobs. Your efforts and kindness to me were wonderful and made me come back with smiles on treatment day.

To Jane Mitchell Thibault: Your regular and thoughtful words of care, prayer, and positivity knows no bounds. You are a mind reader, sending uplifting texts, magically, on my darkest of days.

To Natalie Abraham: Your efforts organizing all of the piles of food from the "Guitar Ladies food train" during hysterectomy week was so very thoughtful and helpful. Having to think through meal prep as I so painfully struggled would have been dreadful for both Mike and for me. Nourishment from all the wonderful food made a huge difference in how I felt physically and emotionally, and to you we are grateful.

To Marianne Peryer: Your check-ins, your visits, and organizing, implementing the amazing Healing Garden have given me a newfound strength and a joy that will last for years to come. I am honoured to call you friend.

To Dr. Karen Anderson: My friend, my confidante, and my adviser. The hours you generously gave me in medical advice and reassurance will never be forgotten; you provided me with much peace of mind. You are so very gracious and thoughtful; your cards, your soups, and your efforts and plants in my garden will be cherished for a lifetime.

To Sue Volcko: Your friendship during this year got me through many tough hours. I have lost count of the number of times you came to the hospital in both emerg and admissions. Bringing me dinners, cards, surprise gifts, my Healing Garden sign, and so much more truly made my year much more tolerable. The sleepovers on radiation treatment days and the numerous drives back and forth made things so much easier, complete with your treats of wine gums and chocolate. If I am Thelma, you are Louise.

To all of my Guitar Ladies: The casseroles, the plants, the knitted socks, the amazing gift baskets full of magazines, candles, blankets, food, and cards—all of you have given me the kind of support that has nourished me and kept my focus toward the finish line. Thank you each and every one for all of your efforts. Truly you have been much, much more than just guitar students. Your thousand little things have melded into one giant big thing for me. And, by the way, get practicing.

To Auntie Emily and Cousin Jenny: You have both been through the ringer, and even though this was all way too close to home, you still sent me encouragement and care. I am blessed.

To Shanny, Tracy, Sue, Mong-Diep, and Sherri: Twenty-five years of friendship. It has been so comforting to me having you all in my life. Thank you for being there when I needed the cheering up and to just attempt to feel normal. It was so hard to lose a year with all of you and harder still to feel like all you ever heard from me were the complaints, the pain, and the discouragement, yet you kept up for me. The melon massages, the organized check-ins, and your attention to the number of texts and visits was all well thought out. Thank you for the coffees, teas, lattes, soups, and shepherd's pie. (Sherri, that naughty gift you brought back from Greece was the best laugh yet.) Time to party!

To my big sissy, Lara: What can I say? Three trips home from California to Nova Scotia in the span of eight months to care for me and to cheer me on. You have been my bodyguard and my watchdog my entire life. Your homemade soups, your carrot cake on my birthday, the cancer-free cookbooks, the pink cashmere poncho and the boxing gloves, the sleepovers, the bonding with Mike and Duey, our midnight giggles after eating "the chocolate," the hilarious "energy-release" day that left me laughing oh so hard have all filled my heart with joy. You are a treasure, a friend, a confidante, and you are all mine. I am glad we finally got to spoon in bed without kicking each other—it only took forty-five years!

To my dear dad: Thank you for rescuing me when I needed it. I am so glad you finally got your boxes all sorted! Now you can start enjoying your remaining years with me. "Every day, in every way, I am getting better and better."

To my dear mother: No mother wants to experience what you went through with me, the angst and worry of a daughter with cancer, and even though your own body was challenging you almost every day, you were still there for me, showing up to put cream on my feet, to hold my hand, to tuck me in, and to pray over me. I am grateful for your love. You must've been an awesome nurse in your heyday.

To our beloved mastiff, Duey: You knew I was sick before any of us. Your furry, velvety, bowling-ball head on my abdomen every night for a year was such a great comfort. I am sorry if I wrecked your sleep over and over again with all of my tossing and turning. Your goofy ways and your amazing warmth and snuggles will be cherished for as long as I live. Thank you also for being friendly to all of the people coming and going in the house; I know that was a challenge given your nature as a guard dog. I wish I could clone you into a million other Dueys.

To my two dear, amazing, darling daughters, Annie and Maddie: There are not words big enough to express the love I have for you. The support you have shown me throughout this journey has been simply incredible. To know I was ill with such a scary disease was just so awful for you both. I know how worrisome the year was, and yet you two continued to amaze me with your smiles, your bravery, and your "wise beyond your years" words. You two are irreplaceable. Watching how you have navigated through all of this and how you have both grown even more as young adult women is breathtaking. I love your strength, your knowledge, and your wonderful ideas.

And lastly, to my One and Only, my dear, sweet hunny-bunny, my hero, my Bubsie, my husband, Michael John Ritcey: Ritz, words are insufficient to fully express my love and gratitude for you. I hope the chapter dedicated to you can provide an inkling into the true love and joy and complete happiness I feel from being with you each and every day, no matter how tough, and no matter what. Thank you for being you. You are the pea in my pod.